EMBOLIC DISEASES - UNUSUAL THERAPIES AND CHALLENGES

Edited by **Michael S. Firstenberg**

Embolic Diseases - Unusual Therapies and Challenges

http://dx.doi.org/10.5772/65590
Edited by Michael S. Firstenberg

Contributors

Roza Chaireti, Katarina Bremme, Xingshun Qi, Andrea Mancuso, Milena Nikolova, Marta Baleva, Petar Krasimirov Nikolov, Ismet Gavrankapetanovic, Adnan Papovic, Mehmed Jamakosmanovic, Elvir Baždar, Lejla Tafro, Stanislaw P. Stawicki, Fabian Giraldo, Bojan Biocina, Fayaz Ahmed, Ahmed Elsayed Mahmoud, Michael S Firstenberg

Published by InTech
Janeza Trdine 9, 51000 Rijeka, Croatia

Notice

Publishing Process Manager Dajana Pemac
Technical Editor SPi Global
Cover InTech Design team

First published June, 2017
Printed in Croatia
Legal deposit, Croatia: National and University Library in Zagreb

Additional hard copies can be obtained from orders@intechopen.com

Embolic Diseases - Unusual Therapies and Challenges, Edited by Michael S. Firstenberg
p. cm.
Print ISBN 978-953-51-3235-6
Online ISBN 978-953-51-3236-3

For EU product safety concerns:
IN TECH d.o.o., Prolaz Marije Krucifikse Kozulić 3, 51000 Rijeka, Croatia,
info@intechopen.com or visit our website at intechopen.com.

Meet the editor

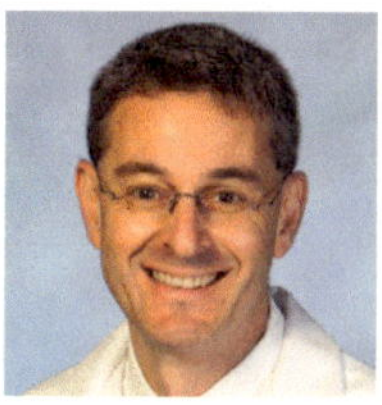

Dr. Michael S. Firstenberg is a board-certified thoracic surgeon actively practicing adult cardiac surgery at the Summa Akron City Hospital in Akron, Ohio. He serves as an assistant professor at Northeast Ohio Medical University. He attended Case Western Reserve University for Medical School, received his general surgery training at University Hospitals in Cleveland, and completed a fellowship in thoracic surgery at the Ohio State University. He also obtained advanced training in heart failure surgical therapies at the Cleveland Clinic.

Extracorporeal membrane oxygenation has always been his passion. He has lectured worldwide and written >100 peer-reviewed articles—many related to ECMO. In addition, he is active in numerous professional societies, clinical research projects, and various quality, process improvement, and multidisciplinary committees.

Contents

Preface

The management of embolic complication of common medical problems represents a significant and ever-evolving medical challenge. The primary focus of this text is to discuss the spectrum of problems that can range from unusual embolic problems in a general population to the specific nuances of diagnosis and management of more commonly observed problems in specific patient populations.

Clearly, the most commonly encountered medical problem that is associated with embolic complications is atrial fibrillation. The management of atrial fibrillation has changed dramatically over the recent years due to the development of diagnostic risk assessment tools, safer and innovative anticoagulation options (i.e., novel anticoagulations), invasive therapies for the treatment of atrial fibrillation (i.e., surgical or catheter-based ablations), and interventions to reduce the risk of embolic complications (i.e., left atrial appendage ligation or closure devices) or the pathologic impact of such complications when they do occur. The management of atrial fibrillation has served as a paradigm for the management of other types of embolic issues. However, it is important to consider that there are a variety of medical problems—including iatrogenic misadventures—that can cause embolic complications. Some of these problems are rare and unusual, and often there is little in terms of randomized trials or extensive clinical literature to guide management. The goal of some of these chapters is to recognize the lack of a standardized approach to the diagnosis and management of some of the less common problems while highlighting some of the existing experiences, data, and options to help guide decision-making and therapy.

Furthermore, it is also critical to recognize that unusual embolic complications can result from specific physiologic conditions—such as during and after pregnancy—or as a consequence of routinely performed procedures—such as orthopedic surgery. Because of patient-specific characteristics and comorbidities, the diagnosis and management options might be substantially different than a population as a whole. Concepts such as prevention, awareness, and early and aggressive treatment reflect the cornerstones to good outcomes. As such, this text will also address some of the unique and challenging aspects in dealing with these specific patient populations and their disease-specific problems.

It is also important to recognize that the diagnosis and management of embolic complications and the pathologic conditions that cause them is an extremely diverse and complex area of medicine. By no means is this text inclusive of all aspects of this challenging and evolving phenomenon, but rather it serves to highlight some unusual problems to help clinicians better understand the broad depth and scope of embolic diseases—and how often the diagnosis and management is much more complex than just a single therapy, like anticoagulation. A common theme throughout this text is that sometimes, while controversial, invasive or surgical options should be considered early for acute or chronic embolic complications.

Probably the most important concept is that embolisms can often be a manifestation of a much more complex or serious medical condition. Without a doubt, such problems—especially in terms of prevention, diagnosis, and management—require an integrated multidisciplinary team to help coordinate care. As with many problems in medicine, such a coordinated team approach must consist of a full spectrum of disciplines and expertise focused on the ability to assess and manage complex problems in a timely and efficient manner. As some of the chapters emphasize, prevention is crucial—especially in various high-risk patient populations. However, since embolisms can occur at any time—and they can present with immediate life or organ-threatening problems (such as neurologic events or limb-threatening ischemia)—dedicated response teams must be organized in advance and be able to respond immediately.

Embolisms, by definition, are pathologic and often associated with severe and potentially fatal complications. This text will hopefully serve as a guide to some of the more challenging and unusual patient populations and problems that occur when medical teams encounter embolic complications. The primary goal of this text is to emphasize the importance of a timely, efficient, and multidisciplinary approach to patient management to achieve optimal outcomes.

Thank you.

Michael S. Firstenberg, MD, FACC
Director, Adult ECMO Program
Associate Professor of Surgery and Integrative Medicine
Northeast Ohio Medical Universities
Department of Surgery (Cardiothoracic)
Akron City Hospital—Summa Health System
Akron, Ohio, USA

Chapter 1

Introductory Chapter: Embolic Diseases - Unusual Therapies and Challenges

Michael S. Firstenberg

Additional information is available at the end of the chapter

http://dx.doi.org/10.5772/intechopen.68936

1. Introduction

Embolic problems are a well-established cause of substantial morbidity and mortality. The challenging aspect of management is recognition of the multi-factorial events that ultimately result in an embolic problem. First and foremost in management is often the acute events that bring the patient to medical attention. While such events, in themselves, can be dramatic in their morbidity and/or mortality—and, therefore, require immediate attention—emphasis must also focus on the precipitating factors that precipitate the embolism. When possible, and reasonable, it is important to identify the source of the embolism, the destination (or destinations) of the embolic material, and the characteristics that might have contributed to the development of the primary source. Management is often structured around controlling the embolism and its clinical consequences.

2. Principles of care

One of the most common thrombo-embolic complications is stroke. Cerebrovascular consequences can span the spectrum of clinical presentations from events that can be minor, self-limited, and potentially asymptomatic events to those that are catastrophically debilitating or fatal. Common causes include thrombotic material from a cardiac source—typically clots from the left atrial appendage in patients with atrial fibrillation [1]. Other cardiac sources include left ventricular thrombus in patients with significant wall motion abnormalities or apical aneurysms/dysfunction in the setting of previous myocardial infarctions or a depressed ejection fraction, infectious sources from endocarditis (also typically intra-cardiac), paradoxical emboli from intra-cardiac shunts (such as a patent foramen ovale), and less common cardiac causes—including benign and malignant tumors [2]. While much energy is focused on cardiac source and systemic effects, it is critical to recognize that there are many others—and often less common or unusual causes. In addition, the foundations for embolic therapy include [3]:

(1) Anticoagulation or anti-platelet therapies to potentially minimize the impact of the initial event.

(2) Interventions—either pharmacologic or mechanical to try to dissolve or remove the distal embolism.

(3) Control or management of the primary source to reduce the risks for recurrence.

(4) Long-term therapies to control the circumstances that resulted in the initial primary sources.

Even though neurologic complications tend to be the most fear, it is important to realize that systemic complications to visceral organ (i.e., hepatic, renal, intestinal) and the extremities can be just as morbid or potential fatal [4, 5]. The focus of many chapters in this text is an update and review of some of these unusual embolic sources. While it is important to recognize that many common clinical problems and their treatments, can lend themselves to the development of protocols and guidelines, some of the more uncommon or unusual presentations and problems can present as considerable diagnostic and therapeutic challenges. The purpose of many of the chapters in this text is to review the data and collective experiences of some of the different types of embolic diseases and to serve as a guide to therapy.

3. Project focus

In addition, even though there are extensive reviews of some of the more common embolic problems—such as left atrial appendage clots, stroke in the setting of either cardiac or non-cardiac sources, and the diagnosis and medical management of the full spectrum of acute and chronic pulmonary thromboembolic disease, these important clinical topics are not considered, other than rarely discussed surgical management, in the contents of this book. The reasons for their exclusion are simple—each topic can clearly be a book in outright (and there are already entire texts devoted to each topic) and even a basic review would overwhelm the primary purpose of this project. Furthermore, the fields in these areas are changing so quickly in terms of diagnostic tools, medical therapies, interventional options, and the standards of care and professional society guidelines that inclusion of some of those topics would only quickly result in an out-of-date reference [6]. Nevertheless, there are some principles that are evolving in the management of embolic disease that are comment regardless of the etiologies. The common principles are echoed as themes throughout this text, but warrant specific discussion.

4. Team-base care

As with many other contemporary disease management guidelines—such as cancers and structural heart disease—the focus is on a multi-disciplinary team approach to the diagnosis and management [7, 8]. The purposes and goals of a team approach should be inherently obviously, but developing and maintaining them often requires substantial leadership in bringing together various disciplines with a patient-centered focus. Professional and disease centric "silos" and traditional models of patient care, including sometimes one-way, fragmented, and ill-coordinated referrals have evolved in the team-based care. Often such teams will have a coordinator—aptly called a "navigator"—whose primary purpose is to help navigate and coordinate the care of the individual patients [9]. As with all journeys, the Navigator will ensure a safe and effective travel, through what is often a complex and challenging path from initial diagnosis to cure. While a Navigator might not be the first healthcare provider a patient encountered when entering into a disease management process, they ultimately serve as the focal point person for care. Even as a patients is individually evaluated by members of the Team, internal referral to the Navigator can help organize the clinical data and help track and coordinate a management plan. Navigators can arrange for testing and follow-up appointments to help not only insure a timely and efficient work-up, but also insure that team-defined care plans are maintained. Typically, a Navigator will help compile all of the relevant diagnostic testing, including critical components of the history and physical exams and provide a framework such that each patient's unique presentation is discussed in a timely manner by all of the disciplines represented by the team. Disciplines represented on such teams can vary, but are often comprised of the core specialties that traditionally manage either the organ systems or the diseases in question. However, there are some key disciplines that often serve as critical team members:

1. Medical specialists (i.e., cardiologists, pulmonologist, oncologists).
2. Surgical specialists (i.e., oncologic surgeons, cardiothoracic surgeons, general surgeons).
3. Therapy-specific specialists (e.g., interventional cardiology/radiology, radiation/medical oncology).
4. Palliative care and hospice medicine.
5. Primary care, hospitalists, or geriatric specialists.
6. Imaging specialists.
7. Advanced practice healthcare providers (e.g., nursing, respiratory therapy, pharmacy, perfusionists, imaging technicians)

In addition, such teams need to be open to all healthcare providers who would be interested in attending and participating. Additional specialists, in specific cases, should be asked to participate to lend their expertise and insights when patients present with a more advanced set of circumstances—such as a nephrologist might be asked to participating in the discussion of a patient who also immunosuppressed from a kidney transplant, or a neurologist and infectious disease experts might be called upon to discuss a patient with a stroke from infectious endocarditis. The overriding principle behind such team-based care is that each case is presented with a focus on evidence based medicine guidelines, local or regional experiences or expertise, objective review of all of the key tests, and a unified consensus as to "best" approach to the management of the patient and their problems. The management of a patient with embolic diseases should also follow such a framework. While the acuteness of a presentation and need for immediate or emergent therapy might preclude a "weekly team conference," it should not change from the borrowing of an established institutional structured approach to the problem. A physical or virtual meeting and discussion of the core disciplines can occur at any time, and hopefully with an existing algorithm in place for disease triage and manage, such meetings can be arranged and effective care-plans determined at any time—even in the absence of a formal "on-call" schedule provided the members are committed to the principles of such team-based care. The current models that are used for Structural Heart Disease or Acute Pulmonary Embolism Teams, throughout of the scope of this text, are being written about more extensively in the literature and might help provide a structure [10, 11].

Important concepts that represent themes throughout this text are that include:

1. Not all sources of embolic disease reflect in here patient co-morbidities—such as atrial fibrillation, atherosclerotic vascular disease, endocarditis, or deep vein thrombosis—just to name a few common intrinsic causes. Some sources may be initially extrinsic to the patient or iatrogenic, such as retained foreign bodies (e.g., guide wires lost during central line placement) or objects that erode into the vascular system after trauma (i.e., bullet fragments).

2. However, it is important to also realize—as emphasized in several chapters—that the pathophysiologic consequences of several chronic disease states, such as liver and renal disease, might predispose patients to increased risks for complex embolic problems. An understanding of the complex biology is a cornerstone to effective management.

3. Similarly, when evaluating a patient with an embolic problem, it is important to consider that not all embolisms are "organic" in nature. While most embolic material consists of biologic material such as clot, atherosclerotic debris, infectious material (i.e., vegetations)—or typically, a combination of one or more components, it is important to consider (as mentioned above) that some embolic material might not be organic, or biologic.

4. Another important concept that is addressed in some of the chapters in this text is that management might vary based upon not only the patient's clinical status, but also the nature of the embolic material. While anti-coagulation or anti-platelet agents still represent a cornerstone to treatment of most embolic complications with the underlying principle that such therapies might minimize the consequences of vascular occlusion with propagation or worsening thrombotic material, acute or definitive treatment might require more invasive therapies. Several of the chapters in this text outline the role and specific techniques for surgical management of embolic complication. With so much emphasis on therapies that focus on manipulations of the clotting cascade—such as anticoagulation, fibrinolysis, or anti-platelets agents—as with all multi-disciplinary approach to complex problems, surgical management options must be considered.

5. Conclusions

It is important to recognize that when faced with a patient with an embolic complication, management can be complexed. Clearly, early and aggressive diagnostic and therapeutic initiatives are critical to prevent further complications. As with many problems, a multi-disciplinary team approach to care is an evolving foundation that is important for optimizing outcomes. Unusual embolic complications, thought far less common than atherosclerotic or those of an intrinsic cardiac source, must be considered and managed using a similar paradigm of care. It is the fundamental purpose of this text to hopefully outline some of the more unusual causes of embolic diseases and emphasize the experiences and data that can guide therapy.

Author details

Michael S. Firstenberg

Address all correspondence to: msfirst@gmail.com

Department of Surgery (Cardiothoracic), Akron City Hospital – Summa Health System, Northeast Ohio Medical Universities, Akron, Ohio, USA

References

[1] January CT, Wann LS, Alpert JS, Calkins H, Cigarroa JE, Cleveland JC, Conti JB, et al. 2014 AHA/ACC/HRS guideline for the management of patients with atrial fibrillation: Executive summary: A report of the American College of Cardiology/American Heart Association Task Force on Practice Guidelines and the Heart Rhythm Society. Journal of the American College of Cardiology. 2014;**64**(21):2246-2280

[2] Bang OY, Ovbiagele B, Kim JS. Evaluation of cryptogenic stroke with advanced diagnostic techniques. Stroke. 2014;**45**(4):1186-1194

[3] Powers WJ, Derdeyn CP, Biller J, Coffey CS, Hoh BL, Jauch EC Johnston KC, et al. 2015 American Heart Association/American Stroke Association focused update of the 2013 guidelines for the early management of patients with acute ischemic stroke regarding endovascular treatment. Stroke. 2015;**46**(10):3020-3035

[4] Shahreyar M, Dang G, Bhandari S, Hanif A, Bashir MW Muppidi V, Bhatia A, Sra J, Tajik AJ, Jahangir A. Predicting outcomes in patients with atrial fibrillation and acute mesenteric ischemia. Journal of the American College of Cardiololgy. 2016;**67**(13S): 717-717.

[5] Geller BJ, Giugliano RP, Braunwald E, Murphy SA Hanyok JJ, Jin J, Mercuri M, Antman EM, Ruff CT. Systemic, noncerebral, arterial embolism in 21,105 patients with atrial fibrillation randomized to edoxaban or warfarin: Results from the Effective Anticoagulation With Factor Xa Next Generation in Atrial Fibrillation-Thrombolysis in Myocardial Infarction Study 48 trial. American Heart Journal. 2015;**170**(4):669-674

[6] Catanese L, Tarsia J, Fisher M. Acute ischemic stroke therapy overview. Circulation Research. 2017;**120**(3):541-558

[7] Holmes DR, Rich JB, Zoghbi WA, Mack MJ. The heart team of cardiovascular care. Journal of the American College of Cardiology. 2013;**61**(9):903-907

[8] Taylor C, Munro AJ, Glynne-Jones R, Griffith C, Trevatt P, Richards M, Ramirez AJ. Multidisciplinary team working in cancer: What is the evidence? British Medical Journal. 2010;**340**:c951

[9] Wells KJ, Battaglia TA, Dudley DJ, Garcia R, Greene A, Calhoun E, Mandelblatt JS, Paskett ED, Raich PC. Patient navigation: State of the art or is it science? Cancer. 2008;**113**(8):1999-2010

[10] Lancellotti P, Rosenhek R, Pibarot P, Iung B, Otto CM, Tornos P, Donal E, et al. ESC Working Group on valvular heart disease position paper—heart valve clinics: Organization, structure, and experiences. European Heart Journal. 2013;**34**(21):1597-1606

[11] Kabrhel C, Jaff MR, Channick RN, Baker JN, Rosenfield K. A multidisciplinary pulmonary embolism response team. CHEST Journal. 2013;**144**(5):1738-1739

Chapter 2

Risk Factors, Treatment and Prevention of Venous Thromboembolism During Pregnancy and Postpartum

Roza Chaireti and Katarina Bremme

Additional information is available at the end of the chapter

http://dx.doi.org/10.5772/67709

Abstract

The naturally hypercoagulable state occurring during pregnancy and anatomical changes and changes in the plasma volume are the main reasons for the increased risk of venous thromboembolism (VTE) during pregnancy and puerperium. This risk is particularly enhanced in the presence of thrombophilia and a previous history of VTE. The cornerstone for treating and preventing VTE is low molecular weight heparin (LMWH). There is currently no consensus on the dosing and the need for monitoring treatment with LMWH, and varying protocols are used in different clinics. The risk models used to stratify the risk for recurrence are based on the presence of factors such as previous VTE, familial history and thrombophilia and lead to decisions on the dosing and the duration of thromboprophylaxis. Treatment with LMWH is considered safe and effective, with low incidence of adverse effects (bleeding, osteoporosis, etc.) and recurrence of VTE. The use of direct oral anticoagulants is currently not recommended in this setting, but case series have not indicated increased embryopathy. The lack of international guidelines and large studies underlines the need for collaboration in order to further improve outcomes and patient safety.

Keywords: pregnancy, postpartum, thromboembolism, anticoagulation, thromboprophylaxis

1. Introduction: venous thromboembolism

Venous thromboembolism (VTE) is a relatively common disease with an incidence of 104–183 per 100,000 person-years among persons of European ancestry [1]. The clinical manifestations of VTE are pulmonary embolism (PE) and deep vein thrombosis (DVT), which is most often located in the lower extremities [2]. The incidence for PE and DVT ranges from 29 to 78 and 45 to 117 per 100,000 person-years, respectively [3, 4]. VTE is associated with significant mortality and morbidity. Sudden death is the initial manifestation for about 25% of patients with PE [5], and PE is an independent marker for reduced survival early after its debut [6, 7]. Around 20–50% of patients with DVT will develop post-thrombotic syndrome [8] with the symptoms varying from mild pain and swelling to severe venous insufficiency and ulcerations [9, 10]. About 5% of the patients with PE can develop chronic thromboembolic pulmonary hypertension, leading to reduced lung capacity and heart failure [11].

The pathophysiology of VTE is complicated and will not be reviewed here. The basic mechanism behind the pathogenesis of VTE is likely attributed to the so-called Virchow's triad: (i) changes in blood flow (i.e. stasis), (ii) vascular endothelial injury and (iii) changes in blood components (i.e. inherited or acquired hypercoagulable states, thrombophilia) [12].

Venous thromboembolism is a multifactorial disease. The risk for VTE increases in the presence of acquired and inherited risk factors, such as thrombophilia [13], immobilization, trauma, recent surgery, cancer, etc. [14, 15]. Additionally, the female sex hormones, predominantly oestrogen, affect the coagulation cascade, tipping it towards hypercoagulability and therefore increasing the risk for thrombosis [16]. For example, the use of combined oral contraceptives [17] and hormone replacement therapy [18] are well-established risk factors for venous thrombosis, especially if other risk factors are present. Pregnancy is a naturally hypercoagulable state, and the risk for thrombosis is increased throughout pregnancy and persisting through puerperium [19, 20]. VTE is the seventh leading cause of maternal morbidity and mortality in Western countries [21, 22], accounting for ca. 10% of all maternal deaths [23]. Considering the burden of the disease and its impact on maternal and foetal health, it is imperative to early recognize and effectively treat venous thrombosis during pregnancy and postpartum. In this chapter, we describe the mechanisms behind the increased thrombotic risk during that period, as well as the principles of treatment and prevention of VTE.

2. Risk factors for venous thromboembolism

2.1. Pregnancy as a hypercoagulable state

During pregnancy, the coagulation balance leans towards hypercoagulability, as a means to protect the woman from fatal bleeding in the case of a miscarriage and during labour. This is mediated mainly by an increase in most procoagulant factors and a decrease in some anticoagulant factors, as well as a decrease in fibrinolytic activity [24].

The levels of fibrinogen begin to increase during the first trimester, reaching profoundly high levels during late pregnancy [25]. Along with fibrinogen, coagulation factors II, VII, VIII, X, XII and XIII increase by 20–200% during pregnancy [26]. Factors V and IX are slightly increased during normal pregnancy or unchanged according to some studies [25, 26]. Factor XIII increases at the beginning of pregnancy and decreases gradually afterwards, reaching levels about 50% of the normal non-pregnant value at term [25]. Factor XI is the only coagulation factor that decreases during pregnancy, with average values at about 60–70% of its normal value (non-pregnant) [25, 27]. Von Willebrand factor increases during pregnancy. During the first half of the pregnancy, it follows the increase in factor VIII, but thereafter increases disproportionally, increasing the ratio of von Willebrand factor antigen to factor VIII coagulant activity from one to about two [25, 28]. Tissue factor does not change during pregnancy [29]. The anticoagulant protein S decreases during pregnancy; this decrease is particularly evident when measuring free protein S and less evident when measuring total protein S. The decrease in protein S persists up to at least 8 weeks postpartum [30]. Protein C remains unchanged [31], but pregnancy induces acquired activated protein C (APC) resistance [32]. Antithrombin values have previously been regarded as virtually unchanged, but later studies have shown that they fall to a level of about 20% of baseline levels [33]. Following partus, antithrombin levels fall additionally to 30% below baseline, with the lowest levels noted 12 hours postpartum, and return to normal about 3 days after birth [34, 35]. Tissue factor pathway inhibitor and thrombomodulin increase during pregnancy [36, 37].

Pregnancy is characterized by hypofibrinolysis. Fibrinolytic inhibitors such as thrombin activatable fibrinolysis inhibitor (TAFI) and plasminogen activator inhibitor-1 (PAI-1), and PAI-2, which is practically non-existent outside of pregnancy, increase [38]. In particular, PAI-1 levels increase significantly due to production from endothelial cells of the placenta and decidua [27, 30].

Plasminogen and tissue-type plasminogen activator increase [39]. The urokinase-type plasminogen activator is also increased during normal pregnancy [40]. Thrombin cleavage products such as D-dimer and fibrin monomers increase, suggesting ongoing and active coagulation [41, 42].

Platelet counts remain within the range of normal values in most pregnancies but can be lower in about 5% of pregnancies (gestational thrombocytopenia) [43, 44], whereas the mean platelet volume is unchanged [45] or increased [46]. Gestational thrombocytopenia is usually mild and occurs during the third trimester. It resolves spontaneously following delivery and platelet counts continue to increase for the first 3–4 weeks postpartum as a marker for increased inflammatory activity. Thereafter, platelet counts return to normal values [47]. Although increased platelet aggregation has been reported during pregnancy [48], the issue of increased platelet activation in an uncomplicated pregnancy is still controversial [49, 50].

Following delivery, there is increased inflammatory activity; C-reactive protein, fibrinogen, antithrombin and platelet counts increase during the first week postpartum [27]. Blood coagulation returns to normal in the first 6–8 weeks postpartum [30, 35].

2.2. Other risk factors for thromboembolism

Along with the haemostatic changes mentioned in Section 1.1, increased venous capacitance and compression of large veins, such as inferior vena cava and iliac vein, by the growing uterus cause stasis [51] and additionally increase the thrombotic risk.

In addition to pregnancy-specific factors, the thrombotic risk increases in the presence of other elements such as thrombophilia. Both acquired (antiphospholipid syndrome) and inherited (such as factor V Leiden, prothrombin gene mutation G20210A, protein S deficiency, protein C deficiency, antithrombin deficiency) thrombophilic conditions are among the factors taken into consideration when calculating the individual thrombotic risk [52–54]. The grade to which these factors contribute varies depending on the specific thrombophilia. There is also evidence that women with thrombophilia have a greater risk of pregnancy complications such as placental abruption, pre-eclampsia, foetal growth restriction, stillbirth and possibly recurrent miscarriage [55].

Other factors that increase the risk for thrombosis, in both pregnant and non-pregnant population, are a medical history of previous VTE, positive familial history for VTE, immobilization, obesity, etc. [56]. Some of those factors are very important when stratifying the individual risk for VTE during pregnancy and deciding on appropriate treatment strategy.

3. Venous thromboembolism in pregnancy and postpartum

3.1. Incidence and type of venous thromboembolism

The risk for VTE during pregnancy is increased, with rates varying from 4 to 50 times higher than in the non-pregnant population. However, despite the increased risk for VTE during pregnancy, the incidence is rather low. In the United States, venous thrombosis occurs in about 1 in 500–2000 pregnancies [57, 58], with DVT being 3–4 times more usual than PE [19, 59]. In Europe the incidence is about 0.71 per 72,000 deliveries, with two-thirds occurring prenatally and the remaining one-third postnatally [60]. The risk for VTE is most pronounced during the postpartum period. Most studies show that the antenatal risk for DVT is equally distributed among the three trimesters [57, 58, 61], whereas PE occurs more often (up to 60%) 4–6 weeks postpartum [62]. During pregnancy, the thrombotic risk is additionally enhanced by the presence of factors such as multiple births, inflammation, infection and diabetes [63, 64]. On the other hand, during the postpartum period, the risk increases in the presence of factors such as caesarean section, obstetric bleeding, pre-eclampsia/eclampsia and infection [20, 64], indicating that the risk factors for thrombosis during puerperium are different compared to the risk factors during pregnancy.

Pelvic vein thrombosis is a rare event outside of pelvic surgery and pregnancy. However, its incidence increases from accounting for less than 1% for all DVT events to 10% of all DVT cases during pregnancy [65]. Additionally, pregnancy-associated pelvic thrombosis is believed to be isolated and not originating from a distal part of the leg [66]. The majority (ca. 90%) of DVT during pregnancy is located in the left leg, probably as a result of the compression of the left iliac artery by the right iliac artery and the inferior vena cava by the growing uterus [58, 67].

3.2. Anticoagulant treatment

Despite the differences in dose recommendations among different committees, the preferred drug for treating VTE during pregnancy is unanimously low molecular weight heparin (LMWH), replacing the previous recommendation on the use of unfractionated heparin (UFH) [68, 69]. LMWH has been shown to cause less bleeding episodes and has a lower risk of causing heparin-induced thrombocytopenia (HIT) and osteoporosis compared to UFH [70, 71]. In contrast to vitamin K antagonists that cross the placenta and can cause teratogenicity, LMWH does not cross the placenta, is easy to administer and has a consistent bioavailability [72]. Fondaparinux does not cross the placenta either, but its use during pregnancy has not been studied extensively; it is primarily recommended for patients with allergy to heparin or HIT [62].

Considering the significant morbidity and mortality associated with VTE during pregnancy and postpartum, prompt diagnosis and treatment of thrombosis is essential to ensure a good maternal and foetal outcome. Although there have not been any major studies on the safety of treating pregnant patients with DVT as outpatients, data from the treatment of non-pregnant patients suggest that this is safe as long as the patient's condition allows it [62]. On the other hand, the safety of treating patients with PE at home, especially on the first days following the event, is more uncertain.

There is no international consensus on the optimal dose for treatment of VTE during pregnancy. LMWH is predominantly eliminated renally, and in the non-pregnant population with a glomerular filtration rate (GFR) of more than 30 mL/min, e.g. no severe renal function impairment, there is no need to adjust the dose or monitor the treatment. However, in pregnant women, due to increased plasma volume and subsequent heparin clearance, as well as weight increase [73], the need for both dose adjustment and monitoring can arise, though expert opinions dissent on that. The initial dose depends on the maternal weight according to the guidelines for non-pregnant patients [69]. The following dosages are recommended for the most commonly used LMWH: dalteparin 200 units/kg once daily or 100 units/kg every 12 hours, tinzaparin 175 units/kg once daily, enoxaparin 1 mg/kg every 12 hours and nadroparin 86 units/kg every 12 hours or 171 units/kg once daily [69]. In Sweden, the recommended start dose of LMWH (dalteparin) is 125 units/kg twice daily or 250 units/kg once daily, since pregnant women need more (25–30%) of LMWH compared to non-pregnant women [74]. The twice-daily protocol is usually preferred in Sweden since clinical observations have indicated a lower bleeding risk.

There is no consensus on whether LMWH should be given once or twice daily, either. Some physicians choose the twice-daily regimen in order to better accommodate the changes in the plasma volume and renal clearance of LMWH during late pregnancy. However, it has been shown [75, 76] that the risk of recurrence does not increase with once-daily anticoagulant regimens in pregnant patients. This, combined with the simplicity of the once-daily treatment and the need for good compliance, makes it an attractive alternative for many physicians and patients.

There are different approaches for the rest of the treatment, following the initial dose, mainly on whether the dosage should be adjusted. In some centres, the dose remains unchanged throughout pregnancy [77]. If an adjustment is deemed necessary, it can be performed either according to the patient's increasing weight [77, 78] or by periodically measuring anti-Xa LMWH levels [69, 73]. The target level is most commonly set to 0.6–1.0 units/mL for a bid regimen and higher for a once-daily regimen, measured 4–6 hours following administration [62]. There are, however, data suggesting that those adjustments are not necessary in most women receiving therapeutic dose of anticoagulants [79–81] showing neither an increase in safety and efficacy of treatment nor a decrease in bleeding complications. The tests currently utilized for the measurement of anti-Xa LMWH are costly and have been reported to be not always reliable [69]. As such, there is no general recommendation on the use of such tests for dose adjustments, but such tests can be useful in patients with renal impairment and extreme low or high body weight [69].

A review by Gandara E et al. [82] on studies where women who were treated with full-dose anticoagulation for up to 6 weeks following diagnosis of VTE (predominantly DVT) and then changed to a dose somewhat lower than 75% of full dose but higher than prophylactic dose, showed that the risk for recurrence was low (ca. 0.65%). In the American College of Chest Physicians (ACCP) Evidence-Based Clinical Practice Guidelines from 2012, dose reduction is named as an alternative approach, especially in patients with high risk of complications, such as osteoporosis and bleeding [62].

Unfractionated heparin can be used as alternative to LMWH in some cases, for example, in patients with severe renal impairment as well as when thrombolysis is considered or when urgent surgery or delivery is planned. When UFH is given, the recommended regimen is twice daily, with doses adjusted to prolong activated partial thromboplastin time (aPTT) into therapeutic range as measured 6 hours following administration [69]. Caution is advised since it is known that aPTT measurement during pregnancy is not as reliable as in non-pregnant patients. The increased levels of factor VIII and of heparin-binding protein observed during pregnancy lead to corresponding decreases in aPPT and increased UFH requirement. It is unclear whether the attenuation in dosage leads to significant bleeding complications [77].

Data on thrombolysis during pregnancy, including data on maternal and foetal safety, is very limited. As such, thrombolytic treatment should be discussed only in the setting of life-threatening PE or in cases of severe DVT where there is a risk of losing a limb [62, 69].

Choosing a delivery option for women on anticoagulation should optimally have been discussed in advance by a multidisciplinary team of coagulation experts, obstetricians and anaesthesiologists. The decision should be based on factors such as the patient's risk profile for both bleeding and thrombosis, the time elapsed since diagnosis of VTE and the actual dosage of anticoagulants, as well as the patient's own preferences. Planned labour induction can be successful in preventing anticoagulation-associated bleedings during partus. In order to ensure patient safety, it is recommended to discontinue anticoagulant treatment 24 hours prior to delivery or neuraxial anaesthesia [62].

The optimal duration of anticoagulation is under discussion. Considering the fact that the increased risk for thrombosis persists throughout pregnancy and puerperium, the current recommendation is that anticoagulation continues for the duration of pregnancy for at least 6 weeks postpartum for a minimum time period of 3 months [62, 69].

3.3. Efficacy and safety of anticoagulant treatment: therapeutic dose

The major adverse effect of treatment with anticoagulants is bleeding. According to the ACCP guidelines from 2012 [62], major nonfatal maternal haemorrhage is defined as a symptomatic bleeding complication into a critical site (intracranial, intraspinal, retroperitoneal, pericardial, etc.), under pregnancy or within 6 weeks postpartum that results in a fall in haemoglobin level of 20 g/L and to transfusion of two or more units of whole blood or red cells [83].

According to a study from 1989, the risk for major antepartum bleeding in pregnant women under anticoagulation with UFH is about 1%, e.g. comparable to the rates noted for non-pregnant patients [72]. LMWH, the drug of choice for treatment and prevention of VTE during pregnancy, has an even milder bleeding complication profile compared to UFH [71, 84]. A review by Greer IA et al. [85] reported bleeding rates of 0.43% (for antepartum haemorrhage) and 0.94% for postpartum haemorrhage (PPH). PPH is defined as blood loss exceeding 500 ml (vaginal delivery) or 1000 ml (caesarean delivery) and is divided into primary PPH, occurring within the first 24 hours after partus, and secondary, occurring between 24 hours up to 12 weeks after partus [86]. Primary PPH has been reported to occur in 1.9% of women receiving treatment dose of anticoagulants [84]. In a study by the authors (unpublished data) on 39 patients with antenatal pelvic vein thrombosis treated with full (adjusted)-dose LMWH, the risk for PPH (<1000 ml) was somewhat increased; however, the risk for severe PPH (>1000 ml) was not increased compared to women without anticoagulation therapy [87], and the rates were comparable to other studies [86]. In the majority of those patients, LMWH was discontinued 24 hours prior to delivery. Knol et al. [86] did not observe an increase in the number of transfused red blood cell units in a population receiving full-dose anticoagulation, suggesting that the majority of observed PPH lacked major clinical significance and the treatment should be deemed safe.

The risk for both HIT and osteoporosis is lower with LMWH compared to UFH [88, 89]. Long-term treatment with UFH has been reported to cause osteoporotic fractures in 2–3% of patients [90], with the rate increasing to 15% in older populations for UFH but being lower for LMWH (3%) [91]. The risk for HIT in patients with UFH has been reported to vary from 0.8% [92] to 2.7% [70] with the respective rates for patients with LMWH being 0% (70). However, antibodies developed in patients with HIT under treatment with UFH have a high risk of cross-reacting with LMWH if such treatment is given [93].

No recurrent thrombosis was recorded for the remainder of their pregnancies in women with pelvic vein thrombosis in the study by the authors mentioned earlier (unpublished data). Similarly, in other studies, the recurrence rates for patients receiving anticoagulant treatment were low [75], indicating a high efficacy of treatment.

4. Thromboprophylaxis in pregnancy and postpartum

The cornerstone of the pharmacological treatment for prevention of recurrent or first-time VTE is LMWH [69]. The grade of the recurrence risk depends on the risk factors for thrombosis, such as previous VTE, thrombophilia and family history, and the patients are treated accordingly.

4.1. Risk stratification for recurrent venous thromboembolism during pregnancy and postpartum

A history of previous thrombosis is the strongest risk factor to predict recurrence risk [94]. Among studies of different designs, the risk for recurrent VTE in women not receiving thromboprophylaxis ranges from 2.4% [95] to 6% [96]. Despite the relatively low recurrence rate, the potentially catastrophic implications of an antenatal or postpartum VTE for mother and foetus have to be considered.

In order to evaluate the risk for thrombotic recurrence and decide on the type of recommended prophylaxis, the patients can be divided into four groups of increasing risk according to the following suggestion: (a) low risk (previous VTE provoked by a transient risk factor), (b) intermediate risk (spontaneous VTE or VTE associated with hormonal treatment or pregnancy), (c) high risk (multiple previous VTE or permanent risk factors for thrombosis) and (d) very high risk (patients with previous VTE and indication for continuing treatment with anticoagulants) [62, 69]. Postpartum (6 weeks following delivery) thromboprophylaxis with LMWH or vitamin K antagonists should be considered for all groups, and the need for additional antenatal prophylaxis should be carefully assessed for groups b–d [62, 69]. These recommendations are subject to change, and the patient can be recommended ante- and/or postpartum prophylaxis depending on the concomitant presence of additional risk factors [68, 69, 97]. If antenatal prophylaxis is given, it should be introduced early upon confirmation of pregnancy [69].

4.1.1. Risk stratification for first-time venous thromboembolism during pregnancy according to family history and thrombophilia

The risk for VTE in individuals with thrombophilia varies, with the highest risk observed on patients with homozygosity for factor V Leiden and prothrombin gene G20210A mutation, whereas the corresponding heterozygotes had considerably lower risks [98]. Familial history of VTE further increases the risk for a first-time thrombosis during pregnancy by two- to fourfold [99].

Similarly to Section 3.1.1, women with thrombophilia and heredity for VTE without previous VTE are divided into different risk groups: (a) women with family history who are homozygous for factor V Leiden or prothrombin gene G20210A mutation, (b) women with family history and all other thrombophilias, (c) women without family history who are homozygous for factor V Leiden or prothrombin gene G20210A mutation and (d) women with all thrombophilias except for those mentioned in (a) without family history. Antenatal and postpartum prophylaxis is recommended for group a, whereas groups b and c are thought to benefit from 6 weeks postpartum thromboprophylaxis. No drug treatment is required for women in group d, unless in the presence of other risk factors, most significantly caesarean section [62, 69]. A special mention should be made to antithrombin deficiency, which is the only other thrombophilia, except for those mentioned in (a) that could warranty antepartum prophylaxis [69].

4.1.2. Risk stratification for first-time venous thromboembolism during pregnancy according to clinical factors

Factors such as BMI > 25 (prior to pregnancy), immobility, caesarean section and co-morbidities (e.g. systemic lupus erythematosus, sickle cell disease) increase the risk for thrombosis independently of the presence of thrombophilia and family history [64, 100]. The extent to which the thrombotic risk is increased by those factors individually is unclear, but is generally considered as modest [62]. However, when antepartum immobility is combined with co-morbidities, the clinician should consider administering thromboprophylaxis during pregnancy and shortly postpartum (7 days) [69].

4.2. Type of thromboprophylaxis

The optimal dose of LMWH thromboprophylaxis is unclear, since studies that compare the different dosages are lacking. For patients with previous VTE who have intermediate or high risk for recurrent thrombosis during pregnancy (see 3.1), it is recommended to use prophylactic or intermediate-dose LMWH. Examples of prophylactic dose LMWH are dalteparin 5000 units subcutaneously every 24 hours, tinzaparin 4500 units subcutaneously every 24 hours, nadroparin 2850 units subcutaneously every 24 hours or enoxaparin 40 mg subcutaneously every 24 hours [62, 96, 101]. Examples of intermediate-dose LMWH include dalteparin 5000 units subcutaneously every 12 hours or enoxaparin 40 mg subcutaneously every 12 hours [62]. The aforementioned dosages can be adjusted depending on body weight and/or renal function [62].

The recommended dose for patients at very high risk for recurrent VTE is higher (adjusted dose or 75% of therapeutic dose) [69]. Adjusted LMWH dose is the dose required in order to maintain a peak level of anti-factor Xa LMWH of 0.2–0.6 units/mL [102] or a trough level of 0.1–0.2 U/ml [103]. For women without a history of VTE who require thromboprophylaxis, it is recommended to administer prophylactic or intermediate-dose LMWH [62]. However, the decision on the optimal dosage is individual, and factors such as risk for complications (bleeding) and patient preferences should be weighed in.

4.3. Efficacy and safety of anticoagulant treatment: prophylactic dose

The risk of bleeding with prophylactic dose of LMWH is generally low and the treatment is considered safe. Most studies in the field do not make a distinction between high- and normal-dose thromboprophylaxis, which makes the results difficult to interpret and the bleeding rates cannot be surely attributed to one type of treatment. In a recent study the bleeding rates were very low according to data derived from 10 studies where the patients were given normal-dose thromboprophylaxis, with overall antepartum rates for severe bleeding (ISTH definition [83]) reported as low as 0% and postpartum rates as 0.3% [104]. In a study by Lepercq et al. that was not included in the meta-analysis in [94], a bleeding incidence of 11.5% was reported; however, in this study, patients with both high and normal prophylaxis doses were included [105]. In a study by the authors, the incidence of bleeding during pregnancy was 12% ($n = 6$) and postpartum haemorrhage had an overall incidence of 20% ($n = 10$) in a cohort of 49 patients treated with high-dose thromboprophylaxis at the Department of Obstetrics and Gynaecology at Karolinska University Hospital in Solna for a time period from 2004 to 2014 (unpublished data). In the same cohort, the incidence of VTE was 2% ($n = 1$, unpublished data). In a study by Pettilä et al. where the patients were treated with normal-dose thromboprophylaxis (UFH or dalteparin), the VTE incidence was 0% [106].

The mean bone density of patients treated with prophylactic doses of LMWH (dalteparin) did not differ from that of patients treated with placebo whereas for patients treated with UFH it was significantly decreased [107]. Similarly, in another study, no difference in bone density was observed between patients receiving prophylactic doses of LMWH and placebo [88]. There are, however, some case reports confirming LMWH-associated osteoporosis [62], and the risk for each patient should be evaluated individually.

5. Future perspectives

5.1. Direct oral anticoagulants

Pregnant and lactating women were excluded from the clinical trials on direct oral anticoagulants (DOAC), e.g. dabigatran, rivaroxaban, apixaban and edoxaban, as there is data suggesting that they may cross the placenta with unclear effects [108]. A recent article [109] identified 233 cases where pregnant women had been exposed to DOAC, with the majority having been exposed to rivaroxaban. The authors did not report an increased risk for embryotoxicity; however, the number of patients was small and the reports were incomplete and diverse [109]. There are currently no guidelines recommending the use of DOAC during pregnancy and breast-feeding.

5.2. Studies

Despite the effectiveness and safety of anticoagulant treatment during pregnancy and postpartum, issues such as the optimal way to adjust and monitor the therapeutic dose of LMWH but also the ideal dose and duration of thromboprophylaxis are yet to be conclusively addressed. Additionally, although there are guidelines from different work groups, differences in local practice remain. There is a need for studies on larger cohorts under international collaborations in order to further advance treatment efficacy and ensure patient safety.

Author details

Roza Chaireti[1,2]* and Katarina Bremme[3]

*Address all correspondence to: roza.chaireti@ki.se

1 Department of Haematology, Karolinska University Hospital, Solna, Sweden

2 Department of Molecular Medicine and Surgery, Karolinska Institute, Solna, Sweden

3 Department of Women's and Child's Health, Karolinska Institute, Solna, Sweden

References

[1] Heit JA, Spencer FA, White RH. The epidemiology of venous thromboembolism. J Thromb Thrombolysis 2016;**41**:3–14. DOI: 10.1007/s11239-015-1311-6

[2] Roussin A Effective management of acute deep vein thrombosis: direct oral anticoagulants. Int Angiol 2015;**34**:16–29

[3] Cushman M, Tsai AW, White RH, Heckbert SR, Rosamond WD, Enright P et al. Deep vein thrombosis and pulmonary embolism in two cohorts: the longitudinal investigation of thromboembolism etiology. Am J Med 2004; **117**:19–25. DOI: 10.1016/j.amjmed.2004.01.018

[4] Heit JA. Epidemiology of venous thromboembolism. Nat Rev Cardiol 2015;**12**:464–474. DOI: 10.1038/nrcardio.2015.83

[5] Poli D, Palareti G. Assessing recurrence risk following acute venous thromboembolism: use of algorithms. Curr Opin Pulm Med 2013;**19**:407–412. DOI: 10.1097/MCP.0b013e328363ed7c

[6] Naess IA, Christiansen SC, Romundstad P, Cannegieter SC, Rosendaal FR, Hammerstrøm J. Incidence and mortality of venous thrombosis: a population-based study. J Thromb Haemost 2007;**5**:692–699. DOI: 10.1111/j.1538-7836.2007.02450

[7] Goldhaber SZ, Visani L, De Rosa M. Acute pulmonary embolism: clinical outcomes in the international cooperative pulmonary embolism registry (ICOPER). Lancet 1999;**353**:1386–1389

[8] Prandoni P, Kahn SR. Post-thrombotic syndrome: prevalence, prognostication and need for progress.Br J Haematol 2009;**145**:286–295. DOI: 10.1111/j.1365-2141.2009.07601

[9] Kahn SR. Post thrombotic syndrome. Hematol Am Soc Hematol Educ Progr 2016; **2016**(1):413–418. DOI: 10.1182/asheducation-2016.1.413

[10] Busuttil A, Lim CS, Davies AH. Post thrombotic syndrome. Adv Exp Med Biol 2017;**906**:363–375. DOI: 10.1007/5584_2016_126

[11] Tapson VF, Platt DM, Xia F, Teal SA, de la Orden M, Divers CH et al. Monitoring for pulmonary hypertension following pulmonary embolism: the inform study. Am J Med 2016;**129**:978.e2–985.e2. DOI: 10.1016/j.amjmed.2016.03.006

[12] Bagot CN, Arya R. Virchow and his triad: a question of attribution. Br J Haematol 2008;**143**:180. DOI: 10.1111/j.1365-2141.2008.07323

[13] Dahlbäck B Advances in understanding pathogenic mechanisms of thrombophilic disorders. Blood 2008;**112**:19–27. DOI: 10.1182/blood-2008-01-077909

[14] Goldhaber SZ. Risk factors for venous thromboembolism. J Am Coll Cardiol 2010;**56**:1–7. DOI: 10.1016/j.jacc.2010.01.05

[15] Heit JA, O'Fallon WM, Petterson TM, Lohse CM, Silverstein MD, Mohr DN et al. Relative impact of risk factors for deep vein thrombosis and pulmonary embolism: a population-based study. Arch Intern Med 2002;**162**:1245

[16] James AH. Prevention and treatment of venous thromboembolism in pregnancy. Clin Obstet Gynecol 2012;**55**:774–787. DOI:10.1097/GRF.0b013e31825cfe7b

[17] Bloemenkamp KW, Rosendaal FR, Helmerhorst FM, Vandenbroucke JP. Higher risk of venous thrombosis during early use of oral contraceptives in women with inherited clotting defects. Arch Intern Med 2000;**160**:49–52

[18] Cushman M, Kuller LH, Prentice R, Rodabough RJ, Psaty BM, Stafford RS et al, Women's Health Initiative Investigators. Estrogen plus progestin and risk of venous thrombosis. JAMA 2004;**292**:1573–1580. DOI: 10.1001/jama.292.13.1573

[19] Kourlaba G, Relakis J, Kontodimas S, Holm MV, Maniadakis N. A systematic review and meta-analysis of the epidemiology and burden of venous thromboembolism among pregnant women. Int J Gynaecol Obstet 2016;**132**:4–10. DOI: 10.1016/j.ijgo.2015.06.054

[20] Kamel H, Navi BB, Sriram N, Hovsepian DA, Devereux RB, Elkind MS. Risk of a thrombotic event after the 6-week postpartum period. N Engl J Med 2014; **370**:1307–1315. DOI: 10.1056/NEJMoa1311485

[21] Lindqvist PG, Torsson J, Almqvist A, Bjorgell O. Postpartum thromboembolism: severe events might be preventable using a new risk score model. Vasc Health Risk Manag 2008;**4**:1081–1087

[22] Chang J, Elam-Evans LD, Berg CJ, Herndon J, Flowers L, Seed KA et al. Pregnancy-related mortality surveillance–United States, 1991–1999. MMWR Surveill Summ 2003;**52**:1–8

[23] James AH, Jamison MG, Biswas MS, Brancazio LR, Swamy GK, Myers ER. Acute myocardial infarction in pregnancy: a United States population-based study. Circulation 2006;**113**: 1564–1571. DOI:10.1161/CIRCULATIONAHA.105.576751

[24] James AH. Pregnancy and thrombotic risk. Crit Care Med 2010;**38**(2 Suppl):S57–S63. DOI: 10.1097/CCM.0b013e3181c9e2bb

[25] Bremme KA. Haemostatic changes in pregnancy. Best Pract Res Clin Haematol 2003; **16**:153–168

[26] Hellgren M. Hemostasis during normal pregnancy and puerperium. Semin Thromb Hemost 2003;**29**:125–130. DOI: 10.1055/s-2003-38897

[27] Hellgren M, Blombäck M. Studies on blood coagulation and fibrinolysis in pregnancy during delivery and in the puerperium. I. Normal condition. Gynecol Obstet Investig 1981;**12**:141–154

[28] Stirling Y, Woolf L, North WRS, Seghatchian MJ, Meade TW. Haemostasis in normal pregnancy. Thromb Haemost 1984;**52**:176–182

[29] Bellart J, Gilabert R, Fontcuberta J, Cerreras E. Miralles F, Cabero L. Coagulation and fibrinolysis in normal pregnancy and in gestational diabetes. Am J Perinatol 1998;**15**:479–486. DOI: 10.1055/s-2007-994069

[30] Kjellberg U, Andersson N-E, Rosén S, Tengborn L, Hellgren M. APC resistance and other haemostatic variables during pregnancy and puerperium. Thromb Haemost 1999;**81**:527–531

[31] Clark P, Brennand J, Conkie JA, McCall F, Greer IA, Walker ID. Activated protein C sensitivity, protein C, protein S and coagulation in normal pregnancy. Thromb Haemost 1998;**79**:1166

[32] Shu H, Wramsby M, Bokarewa M, Blombäck M, Bremme K. Decrease in protein C inhibitor activity and acquired APC resistance during normal pregnancy. J Thromb Thrombolysis 2000;**9**:277–281

[33] James AH, Rhee E, Thames B, Philipp CS. Characterization of antithrombin levels in pregnancy. Thromb Res 2014;**134**:648–651. DOI: 10.1016/j.thromres.2014.07.025

[34] Cerneca F, Ricci G, Simeone R, Malisano M, Alberico S, Guaschino S. Coagulation and fibrinolysis changes in normal pregnancy. Increased levels of procoagulants and reduced levels of inhibitors during pregnancy induce a hypercoagulable state, combined with a reactive fibrinolysis. Eur J Obstet Gynecol Reprod Biol 1997;**73**:31–36

[35] Dahlman T, Hellgren M, Blombäck M. Changes in blood coagulation and fibrinolysis in the normal puerperium. Gynecol Obstet Investig 1985;**20**:37–44

[36] Sandset PM, Hellgren M, Uvebrandt M, Bergström H. Extrinsic coagulation pathway inhibitor and heparin co-factor II during normal and hypertensive pregnancy. Thromb Res 1989;**55**:665–670

[37] De Moerloose P, Mermillod N, Amiral J, Reber G. Thrombomodulin levels during normal pregnancy, at delivery and the postpartum: comparison with tissue-type activator and plasminogen activator inhibitor-1. Thromb Haemost 1998;**79**:554–556

[38] Ku DH, Arkel YS, Paidas MP, Lockwood CJ. Circulating levels of inflammatory cytokines (IL-1 beta and TNF-alpha), resistance to activated protein C, thrombin and fibrin generation in uncomplicated pregnancies. Thromb Haemost 2003;**90**:1074. DOI: 10.1160/TH03-02-0119

[39] Bonnar J, McNicol GP, Douglas AS. Fibrinolytic enzyme system and pregnancy. Br Med J 1969;**3**:387–389

[40] Nakashima A, Kobayashi T, Terao T. Fibrinolysis during normal pregnancy and severe preeclampsia relationships between plasma levels of plasminogen activators and inhibitors. Gynecol Obstet Investig 1996;**42**:95–101

[41] Bremme K, Ostlund E, Almqvist I, Heinonen K, Blombäck M. Enhanced thrombin generation and fibrinolytic activity in normal pregnancy and the puerperium. Obstet Gynecol 1992;**80**:132–137

[42] Chabloz P, Reber G, Boehlen F, Hohlfeld P, de Moerloose P. Br TAFI antigen and D-dimer levels during normal pregnancy and at delivery. J Haematol 2001;**115**:150–152

[43] Matthews JH, Benjamin S, Gill DS, Smith NA. Pregnancy-associated thrombocytopenia: definition, incidence and natural history. Acta Haematol 1990;**84**:24–29

[44] Rouse DJ, Owen J, Goldenberg RL. Routine maternal platelet count: an assessment of a technologically driven screening practice. Am J Obstet Gynecol 1998;**179**:573–576

[45] Howarth S, Marshall LR, Barr AL, Evans S, Pontre M, Ryan N. Platelet indices during normal pregnancy and preeclampsia. Br J Biomed Sci 1999;**56**:20–22

[46] Fay RA, Hughes AO, Farron NT. Platelets in pregnancy—hyperdestruction in pregnancy. Obstet Gynecol 1983; **61**: 238–240

[47] Saha P, Stott D, Atalla R. Haemostatic changes in the puerperium '6 weeks postpartum' (HIP Study)—implication for maternal thromboembolism. BJOG 2009;**116**:1602–1612. DOI: 10.1111/j.1471-0528.2009.02295

[48] Louden KA, Broughton Pipkin F, Heptinstall S, Fox SC, Mitchell JR, Symonds EM. A longitudinal study of platelet behaviour and thromboxane production in whole blood in normal pregnancy and the puerperium. Br J Obstet Gynecol 1990;**97**:1108–1114

[49] Konijnenberg A, Stokkers EW, van der Post JAM, Schaap MC, Boer K, Bleker OP et al. Extensive platelet activation in preeclampsia compared with normal pregnancy: enhanced expression of cell adhesion molecules. Am J Obstet Gynecol 1997;**176**:461–469

[50] Star J, Rosene K, Ferland J, Dileone G, Hogan J, Kestin A. Flow cytometric analysis of platelet activation throughout normal gestation. Obstet Gynecol 1997;**90**:562–568. DOI: 10.1016/S0029-7844(97)00299-8

[51] Gyselaers W, Mesens T, Tomsin K, Peeters L. Doppler assessment of maternal central venous hemodynamics in uncomplicated pregnancy: a comprehensive review. Facts, Views & Vision in ObGyn 2009;**1**:171–181

[52] Hotoleanu C. Genetic risk factors in venous thromboembolism. Adv Exp Med Biol 2017;**906**:253–272. DOI: 10.1007/5584_2016_120

[53] Garcia-Horton A, Kovacs MJ, Abdulrehman J, Taylor JE, Sharma S, Lazo-Langner A. Impact of thrombophilia screening on venous thromboembolism management practices. Thromb Res 2017;**149**:76–80. DOI: 10.1016/j.thromres.2016.11.023

[54] Pengo V, Bison E, Zoppellaro G, Padayattil Jose S, Denas G, Hoxha A et al. APS—diagnostics and challenges for the future. Autoimmun Rev 2016;**15**:1031–1033. DOI: 10.1016/j.autrev.2016.07.028

[55] Alfirevic Z, Roberts D, Martlew V. How strong is the association between maternal thrombophilia and adverse pregnancy outcome? A systematic review. Eur J Obstet Gynecol Reprod Biol 2002;**101**:6–14

[56] Goldhaber SZ, Tapson VF. A prospective registry of 5451 patients with ultrasound-confirmed deep vein thrombosis. Am J Cardiol 2004;**93**:259–262

[57] Marik PE, Plante LA. Venous thromboembolic disease and pregnancy. N Engl J Med 2008;**359**:2025–2033. DOI: 10.1056/NEJMra0707993

[58] Greer IA. Thrombosis in pregnancy: maternal and fetal issues. Lancet 1999;**353**:1258. DOI: 10.1016/S0140-6736(98)10265-9

[59] Heit JA, Kobbervig CE, James AH, Petterson TM, Bailey KR, Melton LJ 3rd. Trends in the incidence of venous thromboembolism during pregnancy or postpartum: a 30-year population-based study. Ann Intern Med 2005;**143**:697–706

[60] McColl MD, Ramsay JE, Tait RC, Walker ID, McCall F, Conkie JA et al. Risk factors for pregnancy associated venous thromboembolism. Thromb Haemost 1997;**78**:1183

[61] Stein PD, Hull RD, Kayali F, Olson RE, Alshab AK, Meyers FA et al. Venous thromboembolism in pregnancy: 21-year trends. Am J Med 2004;**117**:121–125. DOI: 10.1016/j.amjmed.2004.02.021

[62] Bates SM, Greer IA, Middeldorp S, Veenstra DL, Prabulos A-M, Vandvik PO. VTE, thrombophilia, antithrombotic therapy, and pregnancy: antithrombotic therapy and prevention of thrombosis, 9th ed: American college of chest physicians evidence-based clinical practice guidelines. Chest 2012;**141**;e691S–e736S. DOI: 10.1378/chest.11-2300

[63] Simpson EL, Lawrenson RA, Nightingale AL, Farmer RD. Venous thromboembolism in pregnancy and the puerperium: incidence and additional risk factors from a London perinatal database. BJOG 2001;**108**:56–60

[64] Sultan AA, Tata LJ, West J, Fiaschi L, Fleming KM, Nelson-Piercy C et al. Risk factors for first venous thromboembolism around pregnancy: a population-based cohort study from the United Kingdom. Blood 2013;**121**:3953–3961. DOI: 10.1182/blood-2012-11-469551

[65] James AH. Venous thromboembolism in pregnancy. Arterioscler Thromb Vasc Biol 2009;**29**:326–331. DOI: 10.1161/ATVBAHA.109.184127

[66] Chan WS, Spencer FA, Ginsberg JS. Anatomic distribution of deep vein thrombosis in pregnancy. CMAJ 2010;**182**:657–660. DOI: 10.1503/cmaj.091692

[67] Ginsberg JS, Brill-Edwards P, Burrows RF, Bona R, Prandoni P, Büller HR et al. Venous thrombosis during pregnancy: leg and trimester of presentation. Thromb Haemost 1992;**67**:519–520

[68] Royal College of Obstetricians and Gynaecologists (2015) Green-top guideline No. 37a. Reducing the risk of thrombosis and embolism during pregnancy and the puerperium

[69] Bates SM, Middeldorp S, Rodger M, James AH, Greer I. Guidance for the treatment and prevention of obstetric-associated venous thromboembolism. J Thromb Thrombolysis 2016:**41**:92–128. DOI: 10.1007/s11239-015-1309-0

[70] Warkentin TE, Levine MN, Hirsh J, Horsewood P, Roberts RS, Gent M et al. Heparin induced thrombocytopenia in patients treated with low molecular weight heparin or unfractionated heparin. N Engl J Med 1994;**332**:1330–1335. DOI: 10.1056/NEJM199505183322003

[71] Sanson BJ, Lensing AWA, Prins MH, Ginsberg JS, Barkagan ZS, Lavenne-Pardonge E et al. Safety of low-molecular-weight heparin in pregnancy: a systematic review. Thromb Haemost 1999;**81**:668–672

[72] Ginsberg JS, Kowalchuk G, Hirsh J, Brill-Edwards P, Burrows R. Heparin therapy during pregnancy: risks to the fetus and mother. Arch Intern Med 1989;**149**:2233–2236

[73] Barbour LA, Oja JL, Schultz LK. A prospective trial that demonstrates that dalteparin requirements increase in pregnancy to maintain therapeutic levels of anticoagulation. Am J Obstet Gynecol 2004;**191**:1024–1029. DOI: 10.1016/j.ajog.2004.05.050

[74] Essential guide to blood coagulation 2nd edition, 2013. Eds Antovic J, Blombäck M. Wiley-Blackwell, Oxford, UK. ISBN: 978-1-118-28879-5

[75] Voke J, Keidan J, Pavord S, Spencer HN, Hunt BJ, on behalf of the British Society of Haematology Obstetric Haematology Group. The management of antenatal venous thromboembolism in the UK and Ireland: a prospective multicentre observational study. Br J Haematol 2007;**139**:545–558

[76] Knight M, on behalf of UKOSS. Antenatal pulmonary embolism: risk factors, management and outcomes. BJOG 2008;**115**:453–461. DOI: 10.1111/j.1471-0528.2007.01622

[77] Bates SM, Ginsberg JS. How we manage venous thromboembolism during pregnancy. Blood 2002;**100**:3470–3478. DOI: 10.1182/blood-2002-03-0965

[78] Crowther MA, Spitzer K, Julian J, Ginsberg J, Johnston M, Crowther R et al. Pharmacokinetic profile of a low-molecular weight heparin (reviparin) in pregnant patients. A prospective cohort study. Thromb Res 2000;**98**:133–138

[79] Rey E, Rivard GE. Prophylaxis and treatment of thromboembolic diseases during pregnancy with dalteparin. Int J Gynaecol Obstet 2000;**71**:19–24

[80] Smith MP, Norris LA, Steer PJ, Savidge GF, Bonnar J. Tinzaparin sodium for thrombosis treatment and prevention during pregnancy. Am J Obstet Gynecol 2004;**190**:495–501

[81] McDonell BP, Glennon K, McTiernan A, O'Connor HD, Kirkham C, Kevane B et al. Adjustment of therapeutic LMWH to achieve specific target anti-FXa activity does not affect outcomes in pregnant patients with venous thromboembolism. J Thromb Thrombolysis 2017;**43**:105. DOI: 10.1007/s11239-016-1409-5

[82] Gandara E, Carrier M, Rodger MA. Intermediate doses of low-molecular weight-heparin for the long-term treatment of pregnancy thromboembolism. A systematic review. Thromb Haemost 2014;**111**:559–561. DOI: 10.1160/TH13-06-0510

[83] Schulman S, Kearon C, Subcommittee on Control of Anti- coagulation of the Scientific and Standardization Committee of the International Society on Thrombosis and Haemostasis. Definition of major bleeding in clinical investigations of antihemostatic medicinal products in non-surgical patients. J Thromb Haemost 2005;**3**:692–694. DOI: 10.1111/j.1538-7836.2005.01204.x

[84] Romualdi E, Dentali F, Rancan E, Squizzato A, Steidl L, Middeldorp S et al. Anticoagulant therapy for venous thromboembolism during pregnancy: a systematic review and a meta-analysis of the literature. J Thromb Haemost 2013;**11**:270–281. DOI: 10.1111/jth.12085

[85] Greer IA, Nelson-Piercy C. Low-molecular-weight heparins for thromboprophylaxis and treatment of venous thromboembolism in pregnancy: a systematic review of safety and efficacy. Blood 2005;**106**:401–407. DOI: 10.1182/blood-2005-02-0626

[86] Knol HM, Schultinge L, Veeger NJ, Kluin-Nelemans HC, Erwich JJ, Meijer K. The risk of postpartum hemorrhage in women using high dose of low-molecular-weight heparins during pregnancy. Thromb Res 2012;**130**:334–338. DOI: 10.1016/j.thromres.2012.03.007

[87] Bais JM, Eskes M, Pel M, Bonsel GJ, Bleker OP. Postpartum haemorrhage in nulliparous women: incidence and risk factors in low and high risk women. A Dutch population-based cohort study on standard (> or = 500 ml) and severe (> or = 1000 ml) postpartum haemorrhage. Eur J Obstet Gynecol Reprod Biol 2004;**115**:166–172. DOI: 10.1016/j.ejogrb.2003.12.008

[88] Rodger MA, Kahn SR, Cranney A, Hodsman A, Kovacs MJ, Clement AM et al, for the TIPPS Investigators. Long-term dalteparin in pregnancy not associated with a decrease in bone mineral density: substudy of a randomized controlled trial. J Thromb Haemost 2007;**5**:1600–1606. DOI: 10.1111/j.1538-7836.2007.02634.x

[89] Lefkou E, Khamashta M, Hampson G, Hunt BJ. Low-molecular-weight heparin-induced osteoporosis and osteoporotic fractures: a myth or an existing entity?. Lupus 2010;**19**:3–12. DOI: 10.1177/0961203309353171

[90] Douketis JD, Ginsberg JS, Burrows RF, Duku EK, Webber CE, Brill-Edwards P. The effects of long-term heparin therapy during pregnancy on bone density. A prospective matched cohort study. Thromb Haemost 1996;**75**:254–257

[91] Monreal M, Lafoz E, Olive A, del Rio L, Vedia C. Comparison of subcutaneous unfractionated heparin with a low molecular weight heparin (Fragmin) in patients with venous thromboembolism and contraindications to coumarin. Thromb Haemost 1994;**71**:7–11

[92] Girolami B, Prandoni P, Stefani PM, Tanduo C, Sabbion P, Eichler P et al. The incidence of heparin-induced thrombocytopenia in hospitalized medical patients treated with subcutaneous unfractionated heparin: a prospective cohort study. Blood 2003;**101**:2955–2959. DOI: 10.1182/blood-2002-07-2201

[93] Franchini M.. Heparin-induced thrombocytopenia: an update. Thromb J 2005;**3**:14. DOI: 10.1186/1477-9560-3-14

[94] Pabinger I, Grafenhofer H, Kyrle PA, Quehenberger P, Mannhalter C, Lechner K et al. Temporary increase in the risk for recurrence during pregnancy in women with a history of venous thromboembolism. Blood 2002;**100**:1060–1062. DOI: 10.1182/blood-2002-01-0149

[95] Brill-Edwards P, Ginsberg JS, Gent M, Hirsh J, Burrows R, Kearon C et al. Safety of withholding heparin in pregnant women with a history of venous thromboembolism. Recurrence of clot in this pregnancy study group. N Eng J Med 2000;**343**:1439–1444. DOI: 10.1056/NEJM200011163432002

[96] Pabinger I, Grafenhofer H, Kaider A, Kyrle PA, Quehenberger P, Mannhalter C et al. Risk of pregnancy-associated recurrent venous thromboembolism in women with a history of venous thrombosis. J Thromb Haemost 2005;**3**:949–954. DOI: 10.1111/j.1538-7836.2005.01307.x

[97] Mclintock C, Brighton T, Chunilal S, Dekker G, McDonnell N, McRae S et al. Recommendations for the diagnosis and treatment of deep venous thrombosis and pulmonary embolism in pregnancy and the postpartum period. ANZJOG 2012;**52**:14–22. DOI: 10.1111/j.1479-828X.2011.01361.x

[98] Robertson L, Wu O, Langhorne P, Twaddle S, Clark P, Lowe GD et al, for The Thrombosis Risk and Economic Assessment of Thrombophilia Screening (Treats) Study. Thrombophilia in pregnancy: a systematic review. Br J Haematol 2005;**132**:71–196. DOI: 10.1111/j.1365-2141.2005.05847.x

[99] Zoller B, Ohlsson H, Sundquist J, Sundquist K. Familial risk of venous thromboembolism in first-, second- and third- degree relatives: a nation-wide family study in Sweden. Thromb Haemost 2013;**109**:361–362. DOI: 10.1160/TH12-10-0743

[100] Kane EV, Calderwood C, Dobbie R, Morris C, Roman E, Greer IA. A population-based study of venous thrombosis in Scotland 1980–2005. Eur J Obstet Gynecol Reprod Biol 2013;**169**:223–229. DOI: 10.1016/j.ejogrb.2013.03.024

[101] Gates S, Brocklehurst P, Ayers S, Bowler U, Thromboprophylaxis in Pregnancy Advisory Group. Thromboprophylaxis and pregnancy: two randomized controlled pilot trials that used low-molecular-weight heparin. Am J Obstet Gynecol 2004;**191**:1296–1303. DOI: 10.1016/j.ajog.2004.03.039

[102] Ellison J, Thomson AJ, Conkie JA, McCall F, Walker D, Greer A. Thromboprophylaxis following caesarean section—a comparison of the antithrombotic properties of three low molecular weight heparins—dalteparin, enoxaparin and tinzaparin. Thromb Haemost 2001;**86**:1374–1378

[103] Duhl AJ, Paidas MJ, Ural SH, Branch W, Casele H, Cox-Gill J et al, Pregnancy and Thrombosis Working Group. Antithrombotic therapy and pregnancy: consensus report and recommendations for prevention and treatment of venous thromboembolism and adverse pregnancy outcomes. Am J Obstet Gynecol 2007;**197**:457 e1–457 e21. DOI: 10.1016/j.ajog.2007.04.022

[104] Rodger M.. Pregnancy and venous thromboembolism: 'TIPPS' for risk stratification. Hematol Am Soc Hematol Educ Progr 2014;**2014**:387–392. DOI: 10.1182/asheducation-2014.1.387

[105] Lepercq J, Conard J, Borel-Derlon A, Darmon JY, Boudignat O, Francoual C, et al. Venous thromboembolism during pregnancy: a retrospective study of enoxaparin safety in 624 pregnancies. BJOG 2001;**108**:1134–1140

[106] Pettila V, Kaaja R, Leinonen P, Ekblad U, Kataja M, Ikkala E. Thromboprophylaxis with low molecular weight heparin (dalteparin) in pregnancy. Thromb Res 1999;**96**:275–282

[107] Pettilä V, Leinonen P, Markkola A, Hiilesmaa V, Kaaja R. Postpartum bone mineral density in women treated for thromboprophylaxis with unfractionated heparin or LMW heparin. Thromb Haemost 2002;**87**:182–186

[108] Tang AW, Greer I. A systematic review on the use of the new anticoagulants in pregnancy. Obstet Med 2013;**6**:64–71. DOI: 10.1177/1753495X12472642

[109] Beyer-Westendorf J, Michalski F, Tirrl L, Middeltorp S, Cohen H, Abdul Kadir R et al. Pregnancy outcome in patients exposed to direct oral anticoagulants- and the challenge of event reporting. Thromb Haemost 2016;**116**;651–658. DOI: 10.1160/TH16-04-0305

Chapter 3

Surgical Management of Chronic Pulmonary Embolism

Fabian Andres Giraldo Vallejo

Additional information is available at the end of the chapter

http://dx.doi.org/10.5772/67708

Abstract

Chronic thromboembolic pulmonary hypertension (CTEPH) is a rare but life-threatening complication of acute pulmonary embolism (PE). This entity is the consequence of a persistent obstruction of the pulmonary arteries and progressive vascular remodeling. Some patients with CTEPH do not have a history of classic pulmonary embolism symptoms. The diagnostic process to detect CTEPH should include ventilation-perfusion scintigraphy, which has a high sensitive and negative predictive value (nearly 100%) and CT angiography demonstrating typical features of CTEPH (occlusion of pulmonary arteries, mosaic perfusion or intraluminal bands or webs). Patients suspected of having CTEPH must be referred to an experienced center in order to complete the diagnostic workup (right-heart catheterization and pulmonary angiography) and determine the best treatment. Pulmonary endarterectomy (PEA) remains the treatment of choice for CTEPH and is associated with excellent long-term results and a highly curative rate. Patients with inoperable CTEPH are given medical and interventional modalities.

Keywords: thromboembolism, pulmonary hypertension, pulmonary endarterectomy

1. Introduction

Chronic thromboembolic pulmonary hypertension (CTEPH) is caused by a persistent obstruction of the pulmonary arteries after a pulmonary embolism (PE) that has not resolved despite 3 months of medical therapy with anticoagulants and is defined as a raised mean pulmonary artery pressure (at least 25 mmHg at rest), a pulmonary capillary wedge pressure of ≤ 15 mmHg and at least one (segmental) perfusion defect detected by lung scanning, multi-detector computed tomographic angiography or pulmonary angiography [1, 2]. CTEPH is a form of pulmonary artery hypertension (PAH) characterized by the occlusion of the pulmonary arteries by organized fibrotic thrombi leading to increased pulmonary vascular resistance (PVR). The consequential effect is dyspnea, right heart failure and even death. CTEPH is classified as group IV according to the WHO classification of pulmonary hypertension [3]. Some patients may present symptoms and signs of CTEPH but no pulmonary hypertension; this presentation should be termed chronic thromboembolic disease, although the management of these patients does not differ to that of the classic CTEPH patients.

The most common cause of CTEPH is non-resolving acute pulmonary embolism (PE) and can occur after one or multiple episodes. Occasionally, CTEPH may develop after in situ pulmonary artery thrombosis which could be associated with the inflammation of vessel walls [4].

CTEPH can be mistaken for PE; it is important to differentiate between these, in order to diagnose the chronic disease as early as possible. Once the diagnosis of CTEPH is made, careful patient selection in experienced centers is preferable in order to obtain the best results for these patients.

Because of its unique characteristics, CTEPH is the only form of PH that can be curable by pulmonary endarterectomy (PEA); although, this is a complicated surgery and not every patient may be fit to undergo such a procedure. The most benefited patients are those who present a proximal compromise [5].

CTEPH remains underdiagnosed and carries a poor prognosis. Medical and interventional treatment are options for patients that are not surgical candidates. In this chapter, the available information on the surgical treatment of CTEPH is summarized.

2. Historical note

The first description of the CTEPH was made in 1928 by Dr Ljungdahl on two symptomatic patients with chronic obstruction of the pulmonary arteries who ultimately died of right heart failure [6]. The first successful embolectomies for recurrent pulmonary embolism were reported by Allison and colleagues in 1958 and by Snyder and colleagues in 1962 [7, 8]. Then, Cabrol et al. refined the technique using a lateral thoracotomy in order to obtain access to distal pulmonary branches [9]. In 1980, Daily et al. reported the use of cardiopulmonary bypass (CPB) and hypothermic circulatory arrest, allowing the reduction of severe back bleeding and improving the visualization of the pulmonary arteries during endarterectomy [10]. This is the current preferred technique.

3. Morphology

The process of the disease typically occurs in the proximal pulmonary arteries from trunk to sublobar levels. The distal vasculature remains patent. This presentation is the basis for the surgical approach of CTEPH. The disease may develop from a single embolic episode with non-resolution of large thrombi or from repeated thromboembolic episodes [11]. The remaining unobstructed pulmonary arteries are exposed to high flow and eventually high pressure. Then, proximal patent pulmonary arteries enlarge, and the distal arterial vasculature develops changes of pulmonary hypertension such as intimal proliferation and medial hypertrophy. The characteristic diagnostic finding of primary pulmonary hypertension, the plexiform lesion, is also observed in CTEPH [12]. The occlusive process is usually central, incipient and unresponsive to antithrombotic or anticoagulant therapy when the thrombi become fibrotic and endothelialized. The thrombotic material has well-organized fibrous tissues, penetrating blood vessels, elastic fibers and no endothelial cells. The arterial layers demonstrate intimal and medial hyperplasia. Infarction of the lung tissue is rarely observed [2]. These microvascular changes explain why CTEPH is a progressive disease even in the absence of recurrent thromboembolic events.

4. Epidemiology

The estimated prevalence of CTEPH after acute pulmonary embolism is 0.1–4% after 2 years [2, 13–16]. The median age at diagnosis is 63 years, and both genders are equally affected [17]. The risk of developing CTEPH is increased in patients with recurrent venous thromboembolism, echocardiographic signs of pulmonary hypertension at the initial presentation and large perfusion defects. Common risk factors for venous thromboembolism (factor V Leyden, factor II mutation) are not associated with the development of CTEPH except for the presence of antiphospholipid antibodies, which predispose patients to acute venous thromboembolism and CTEPH [1, 18–20]. Different disorders considered to be risk factors include inflammatory bowel disease, splenectomy, myeloproliferative disorders, chronic osteomyelitis and the presence of permanent central venous lines, pacemakers or ventriculoatrial shunts [20–23]. These disorders are associated with chronic inflammation, an increased risk of repeated bloodstream infection or both, which may contribute to the non-resolution of thromboembolic material [1]. C-reactive protein is also implicated in the development of CTEPH [24]. Infection of thrombotic material by blood-borne pathogens could predispose to the development of CTEPH, specially in patients with permanent central venous lines, pacemakers or ventriculoatrial shunts [25].

5. Natural history

It is relatively infrequent to find a complete resolution of pulmonary embolism. If adequate anticoagulation therapy has been done, more than 50% of patients have residual perfusion defects 6 months after the diagnosis of pulmonary embolism [26]. However, the majority of these patients do not develop florid chronic pulmonary hypertension; in fact, patients presenting signs of pulmonary hypertension during an episode of acute pulmonary embolism are unlikely to develop CTEPH, and most of these patients recover a stable phase of right ventricular functions within 40 days [13]. Some patients, however, present persistent pulmonary hypertension and others develop pulmonary hypertension after a symptom-free interval that can last from months to years [14]. Hemodynamic deterioration may be the result of recurrent thromboembolism or in situ pulmonary artery thrombosis. Without intervention, survival is compromised and proportional to the degree of pulmonary hypertension at the time of diagnosis [27, 28]. To remind, pulmonary hypertension is not a feature of acute pulmonary embolism since the right ventricle (RV) is incapable of generating high pressures in early stages. In that order, any patient presenting with acute pulmonary embolism and elevated pulmonary resistances may already have CTEPH. In a study, the 5-year survival rate was 30% among patients with a mean pulmonary pressure > 40 mmHg at time of diagnosis, and it dropped dramatically to 10% among those with a mean pulmonary pressure > 50 mmHg [29]. In another study, a mean pulmonary artery pressure of 30 mmHg marked the threshold for poor prognosis [30].

6. Clinical features and diagnosis

6.1. Symptoms

In general, symptoms do not develop until months or years after the embolic event [2]. They occur as a result of right ventricular failure or pulmonary hypertension. Progressive dyspnea on exertion is the predominant symptom of CTEPH [11]. Additionally, patients might present with fatigue, substernal chest pain with exercise, pleuritic pain and hemoptysis [11, 31].

6.2. Signs

Relevant physical findings are related to right heart failure: jugular venous distention, ascites, hepatomegaly and peripheral edema. The right ventricle may be enlarged and palpable near the lower left sternal border. The pulmonic second sound is accentuated and split. A murmur of tricuspid regurgitation might be heard in severe right heart failure.

CTEPH should be considered in all patients who have an evident history of acute pulmonary embolism. Despite 25% of the patients diagnosed as having CTEPH, there are no documented acute pulmonary embolism events [32]. Thus, CTEPH should be suspected in any patient with otherwise unexplained pulmonary hypertension.

6.3. Diagnostic studies

The chest radiograph may demonstrate right ventricle enlargement and the prominence of central pulmonary arteries. The ECG frequently shows RV hypertrophy with strain, right axis deviation, ST depression, T-wave inversion in the anterior precordial leads and occasionally right bundle branch block [31]. Transthoracic echocardiography provides the initial objective evidence for the presence of PAH. Findings in chronic thromboembolic and other forms of PAH include the enlargement of right cardiac chambers, tricuspid regurgitation as a consequence from this enlargement, the flattening or paradoxical motion of the interventricular septum and impaired left ventricular diastolic filling not caused by primary left ventricular diastolic dysfunction or valvular heart disease [33, 34]. Pulmonary function studies are necessary to exclude restrictive or obstructive pulmonary parenchymal disease as the cause of PAH.

Ventilation-perfusion scanning is the preferred diagnostic tool because of its high sensitivity and a negative predictive value of almost 100% [35]. In that order, CTEPH is practically ruled out if the scan is normal [35]. A lung perfusion scan showing at least one segmental or larger defect is suggestive of chronic vascular obstruction [2]. Often, the scan underestimates the severity of an obstructive disease [36, 37]. Perfusion defects can also occur in other disorders such as pulmonary veno-occlusive disease, pulmonary vasculitis, fibrosing mediastinitis or malignant disease [38–40]. CT scanning and MRI of the chest are important diagnostic tools and are being used with increasing frequency [41, 42]. If imaging suggests the presence of CTEPH, patients should be evaluated with right-heart catheterization to measure the right ventricle and pulmonary artery pressures and to evaluate the presence of shunting at the atrial or ventricular level. Pulmonary angiography is safe in patients with chronic pulmonary hypertension [2, 43]. Typical findings include dilated proximal pulmonary arteries, varying degrees of obstruction of lobar arteries, filling defects, web or bands or thrombosed vessels suggesting the presence of organized thrombi [44]. In order to avoid repeat procedures, angiography should be done in a center that assesses the patient's suitability for surgery. A general screening after acute pulmonary embolism is not recommended, given the low risk of developing CTEPH after such an event [45–47]. Care must be taken, however, in patients who show symptoms after an episode of acute pulmonary embolism. Echocardiography is widely used when suspecting pulmonary hypertension. A diagnostic approach that combines an electrocardiogram with no signs of hypertrophy in the right ventricle and a normal natriuretic peptide (N-terminal-pro-brain-type fragment) has a negative predictive value of 99% for CTEPH [48].

Angioscopy is an alternative tool adjunct to angiography, CT or MRI when these modalities cannot establish the diagnosis properly [49].

7. Treatment

Patients diagnosed with CTEPH should have life-long anticoagulation, even those who underwent successful PEA. The target international normalized ratio is 2.0 to 3.0. The use of filters in the inferior vena cava remains controversial [50]. Currently, the use of these filters is indicated when therapeutic anticoagulation is not feasible or when recurrent venous thromboembolism occurred despite sufficient anticoagulation [51]. Prospective studies on this matter are warranted.

7.1. Surgical selection

The most important criterion that determines whether a patient with CTEPH might be a candidate for PEA is the presence of surgically accessible lesions. PEA should be considered in symptomatic patients who have hemodynamic or ventilatory impairment at rest or with exercise [52]. The decision to proceed with PEA in patients with CTEPH is difficult based on their preoperative pulmonary hemodynamic profile and the anticipated improvement in these hemodynamics postoperatively [27]. The basis for this concern is that the elevated vascular resistance not only arises from central (surgically accessible) vessels but also from secondary, small vessels with arteriopathy [27]. A preoperative approach should differentiate these two components and anticipate the postoperative hemodynamic outcome. This important issue remains relatively subjective. There is a high correlation between the postoperative level of pulmonary vascular resistance (PVR) and mortality. In a study by Jamieson and colleagues including 500 consecutive operated patients with an overall mortality of 4.4%, 77% of deaths were related to residual high pulmonary artery pressures. Patients with a postoperative PVR > 500 dynes-sec-cm^{-5} had a mortality rate of 30.6% compared to 0.9% in patients with a postoperative PVR < 500 dynes-sec-cm^{-5} [53]. The majority of patients who undergo a PEA have a PVR > 300 dynes-sec-cm^{-5}. Experienced centers report a range of preoperative PVR between 700 and 1100 dynes-sec-cm^{-5} [53–58]. Symptomatic patients at the lower end of these values include those with involvement limited to one pulmonary artery, those accustomed to a vigorous activity and those who live at high altitudes [52]. Operations should also be considered for patients with nearly normal pulmonary hemodynamics at rest but marked pulmonary hypertension induced by exercise. The only absolute contraindication to operation is the presence of severe underlying obstructive or restrictive lung diseases [52]. The most important risk factor for surgery is the presence of high pulmonary resistances without visible abnormalities by angiography [53]. Older patients and severe RV failure are associated with increased risk but do not preclude surgery.

7.2. The technique of operation

This is the description of the current accepted and most widely used technique for PEA. Electroencephalographic recording is essential to ensure the absence of cerebral activity before circulatory arrest is induced. The patient's head is involved in a cooling jacket. Standard preparations for the establishment of cardiopulmonary bypass (CPB) are made. A median sternotomy is performed. Cannulas are inserted into the ascending aorta and both venae cavae, which are encircled with tapes. Immediately after CPB starts, cooling is initiated (including the head jacket and the cooling blanket). This could take 45 minutes to 1 hour [59]. A venting catheter is placed in the left atrium through the upper right pulmonary vein. If the patient's condition allows it, autologous whole blood is withdrawn for later use. The deficit can be replaced with a crystalloid solution. The aorta is clamped and cold blood cardioplegia is given. Additional myocardial protection could be done by subsequent infusions of cold cardioplegic solution, every 15 to 20 minutes. During the cooling period, mobilization of the right pulmonary artery from the ascending aorta is made as well as the mobilization of the superior vena cava. Also, methylprednisolone (7 mg/kg) and thiopental (10–15 mg/kg) are administered to favor the neuroprotective effect of hypothermia. Mannitol (0.3–0.4 mg/kg) and furosemide (100 mg) are infused to preserve the renal function. Once the core temperature has reached 12–14°C and the electroencephalogram becomes isoelectric, circulatory arrest is established [60]. Both encircling tapes of superior and inferior vena cava are secured to ensure complete drainage and to avoid air embolization into the venous cannulae during circulatory arrest. An incision is made in the right pulmonary artery between the aorta and the superior vena cava (**Figure 1**), extending the incision toward the right lower lobe artery, a few millimeters farther from the takeoff of the middle lobe artery (**Figure 2**). Using a sharp dissector can help establish an endarterectomy plane (**Figure 3**). The intima and a portion of the media are removed. Establishment of the correct plane is essential—too deep will result in artery perforation, too shallow will result in an inadequate endarterectomy [61]. When the adequate plane is achieved, the layer will dismount easily. The core of the thrombus is dissected in a circumferential manner (**Figure 4**) and removed from each subsegmental branch and from the pulmonary artery (**Figure 5**). Gentle traction with forceps is applied to the core as well as opposite force to the pulmonary wall that will facilitate the removal of the specimen (**Figure 6**). The remaining core is removed from the proximal portion of the right pulmonary artery (**Figure 7**). The arteriotomy is closed with a continuous 5–0 or 6–0 polypropylene suture (**Figure 8**). If needed, a pericardial patch can be used that is sutured into place with a continuous 6–0 polypropylene suture. The period of circulatory arrest ranges from 20 to 25 minutes. Cold blood is reperfused for 8–10 minutes between these intervals. As for the left side, the incision begins in the pulmonary trunk and extends onto the left pulmonary artery to the level of the pericardial reflection (**Figure 9**). Endarterectomy of the left side mirrors that of the right pulmonary artery. The core is removed from the upper lobe artery and each subsegmental branch. The artery is closed in a continuous fashion or with

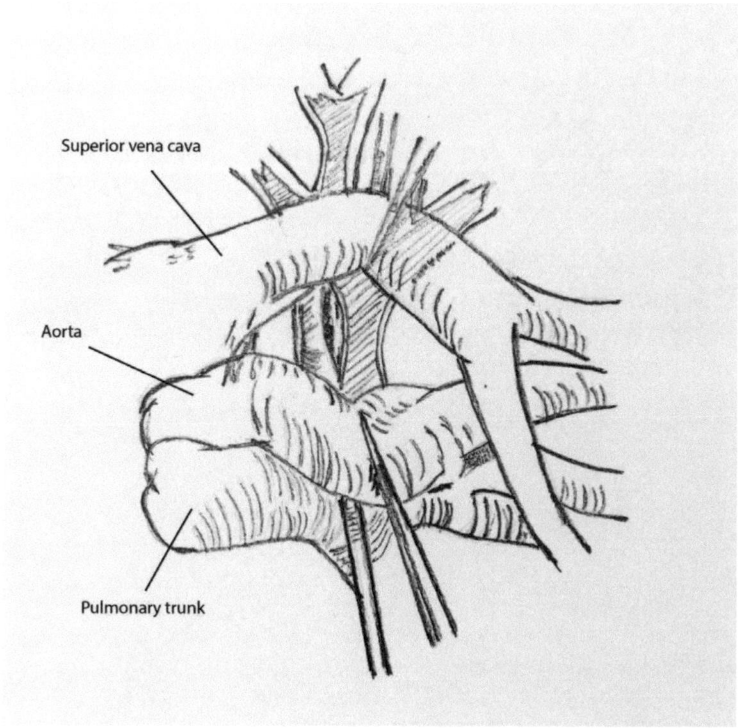

Figure 1. An approach to pulmonary artery. View from left side. Superior vena cava is completely mobilized and retracted laterally, and aorta is retracted medially. The incision on pulmonary artery is done between these two vessels.

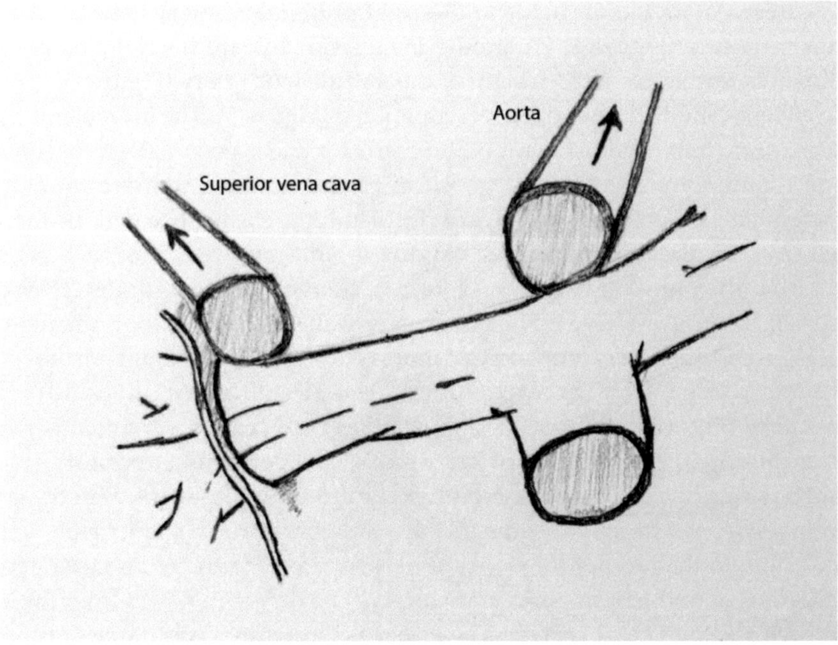

Figure 2. Exposure of distal right pulmonary artery between aorta and superior vena cava. Dashed line indicates line of incision.

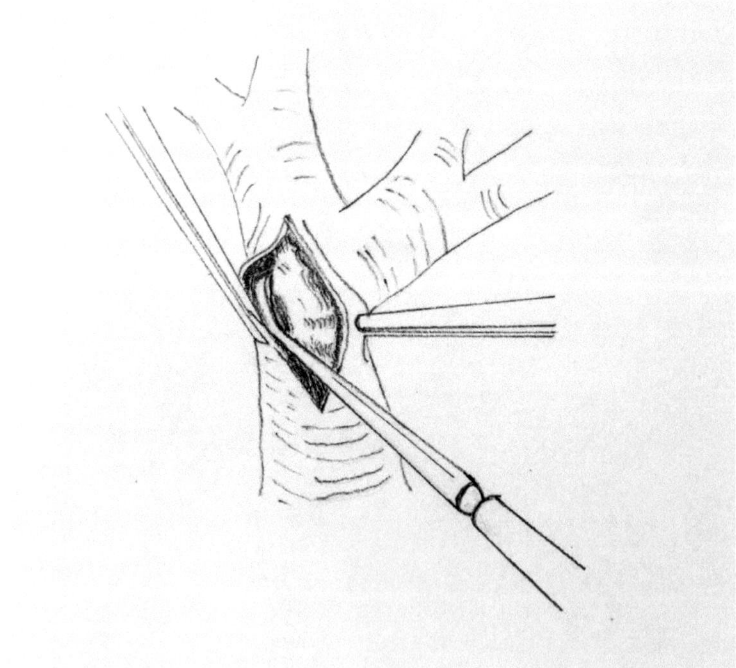

Figure 3. Endarterectomy plane is facilitated with a sharp dissector.

http://dx.doi.org/10.5772/67708

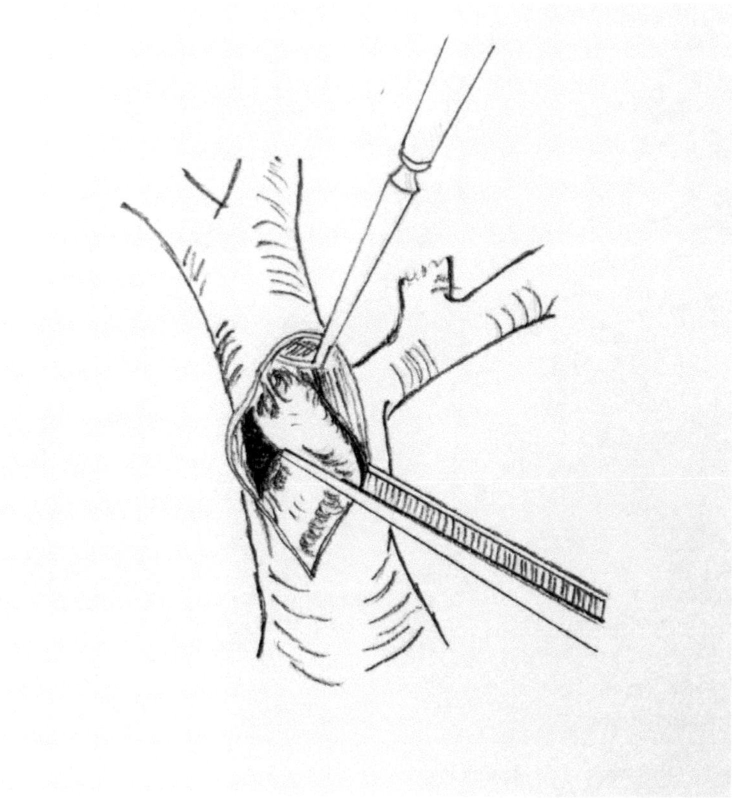

Figure 4. Circumferential isolation of the core of the thrombus and extraction from upper lobe and distal pulmonary artery.

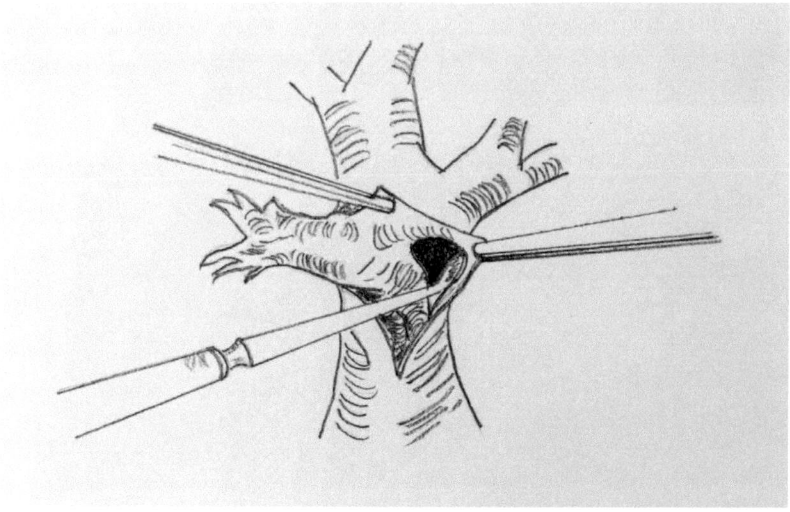

Figure 5. Extraction of the core of the thrombus.

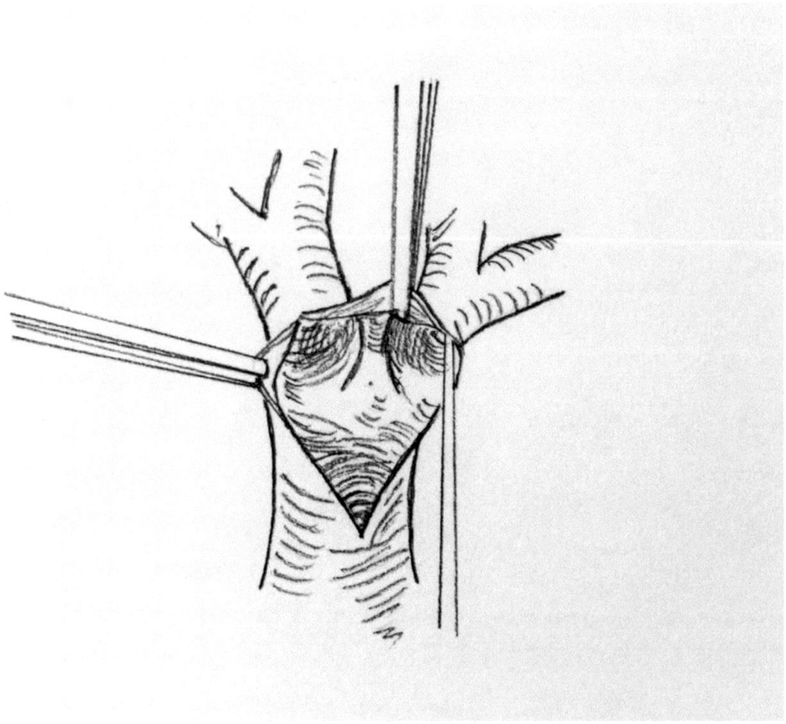

Figure 6. Separation of core from proximal pulmonary artery.

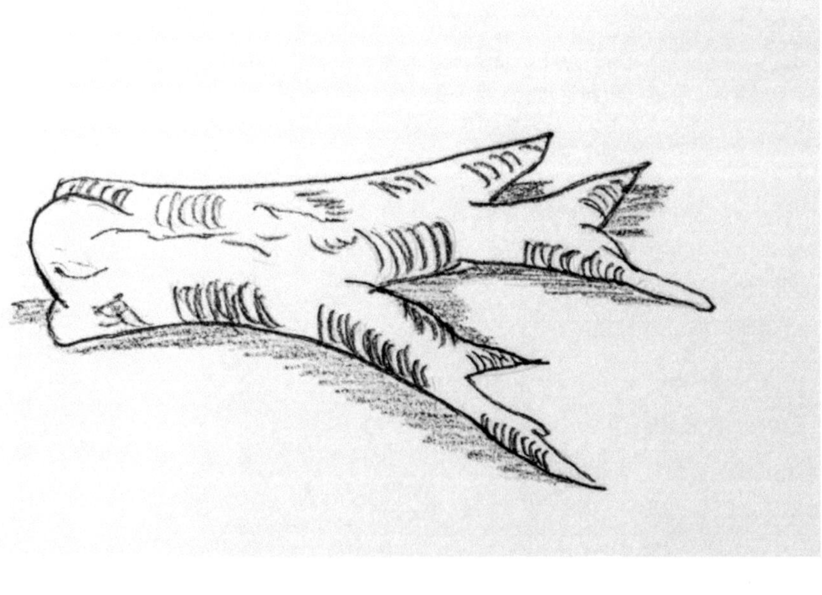

Figure 7. Complete extraction of core specimen.

http://dx.doi.org/10.5772/67708

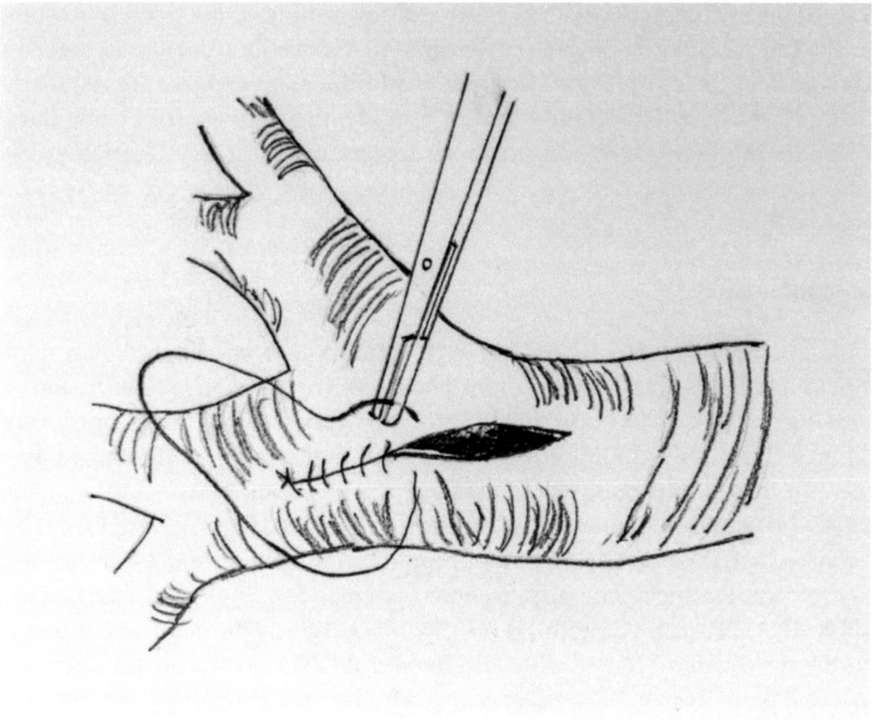

Figure 8. Arteriotomy is closed with a continuous 5–0 or 6–0 polypropylene suture.

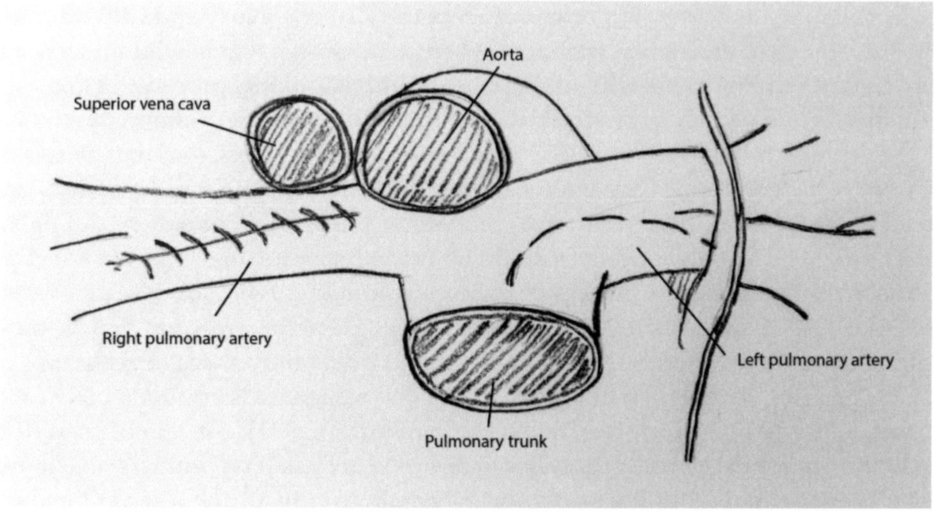

Figure 9. Incision in left pulmonary artery (dashed line) begins in the pulmonary trunk and extends onto the left pulmonary artery.

an autologous pericardial patch. CPB begins and rewarming of the patient is established. If any other defects are present, such as patent foramen ovale or atrial septal defect, these are corrected to prevent the right-to-left shunting. If additional procedures are required, they are made during rewarming [62]. Right ventricle remodeling occurs within a few days, so, any tricuspid regurgitation rarely needs repair or replacement [61, 62]. Deariation maneuvers from cardiac chambers are performed, CPB is discontinued and the procedure is completed in the usual fashion.

7.3. Postoperative care

An FiO_2, high enough to maintain SaO_2 > 95%, during mechanical ventilation, is preferred. $PaCO_2$ should be ≤ 35 mmHg. An important postoperative problem is reperfusion of the pulmonary edema and occurs in approximately 10% of patients [61]. Lung injury can develop within the first 2 days of exhibiting hypoxemia and radiographic infiltrates in areas where endarterectomy has been done [63]. Treatment for this condition includes maintaining a SaO_2 >90% and positive end-expiratory pressures of 5–10 cm. Prostaglandin E1 at 0.01–1 mg/min and inhaled nitric oxide (20–40 parts per million) may be useful. Diuretics use is often required to reduce the incidence of pulmonary edema [64]. Since the reperfusion injury is neutrophil mediated, treatment with agents that block the selectin-mediated adhesion of leucocytes to the endothelium (Cylexyn) could be useful [63]. Extracorporeal support has been used in selected patients with serious reperfusion injury [52]. Permanent anticoagulation with warfarin is started on the second postoperative day [60].

7.4. Results

Experienced centers have a mortality that ranges from 4.4 to 21% [53, 64–68]. Risk factors commonly associated with mortality in the early postoperative period are RV failure related to residual pulmonary hypertension, reperfusion lung injury and CPB duration [10, 52, 53]. Survival rates are almost the same when comparing patients who underwent pulmonary endarterectomy alone with other patients with additional procedures (5.8 vs. 6.7%, respectively) [62]. In the largest study with patients undergoing pulmonary endarterectomy, the 6-year survival rate was 75% (**Figure 10**) [69]. The most common causes of late death were recurrent pulmonary embolism and persistent pulmonary hypertension [69]. Hemodynamic outcomes after pulmonary endarterectomy for most patients are favorable [56, 64–67, 70–74]. The only long-term study on hemodynamics after PEA observed persistent pulmonary hypertension in 24% of patients who had pulmonary vascular resistance of more than 500 dynes-sec-cm^{-5} after 4 years [75]. Dramatic reduction and, sometimes, normalization of the pulmonary artery pressure and pulmonary vascular resistance can be achieved. The mean reduction in pulmonary vascular resistance is approximately 65% [52]. Most patients are in New York Heart Association Functional Classification, class III or IV, before surgery; after the procedure, they can improve to class II or I and are able to resume normal activities [11, 69, 70]. Recurrent thromboembolism requiring a second endarterectomy has occurred in several patients in whom anticoagulation was discontinued or given improperly [76].

http://dx.doi.org/10.5772/67708

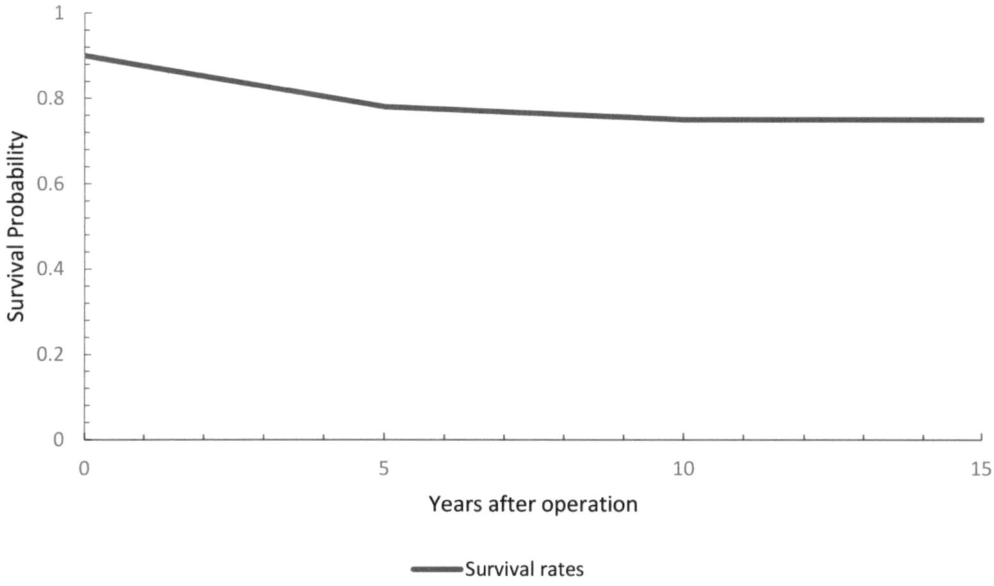

Figure 10. Survival after pulmonary thromboendarterectomy in 532 patients. Adapted from Archibald et al.

8. Conclusions

CTEPH is a life-threatening complication of pulmonary embolism. There are notable differences in the treatment from that of other forms of pulmonary hypertension. A complete diagnostic assessment should be done in those patients with unexplained pulmonary hypertension. These studies should include a ventilation-perfusion scintigraphy, right-heart catheterization and pulmonary angiography. It is recommended though that the final diagnostic and therapeutic approach should be performed in experienced centers.

PEA is the preferred treatment and remains the only potentially curative approach. For patients in whom surgery is not an option, riociguat is the only approved drug that improves hemodynamics and exercise capacity. Balloon pulmonary angioplasty is yet to be proven effective in the treatment of these patients. An increased understanding of the prevalence of this condition and opportunities of surgical cure should benefit a larger volume of patients.

Author details

Fabian Andres Giraldo Vallejo

Address all correspondence to: fabiangiraldomd@gmail.com

Heart Institute of Bucaramanga, Bucaramanga, Colombia

References

[1] Lang IM, Pesavento R, Bonderman D, Yuan JX-J. Risk factors and basic mechanisms of chronic thromboembolic pulmonary hypertension: a current understanding. Eur Respir J. 2013;41(2):462-8.

[2] Moser KM, Auger WR, Fedullo PF. Chronic major-vessel thromboembolic pulmonary hypertension. Circulation. 1990;81(6):1735-43.

[3] Kim NH, Delcroix M, Jenkins DP, Channick R, Dartevelle P, Jansa P, et al. Chronic thromboembolic pulmonary hypertension. J Am Coll Cardiol. 2013;62(25):D92-9.

[4] Egermayer P, Peacock AJ. Is pulmonary embolism a common cause of chronic pulmonary hypertension? Limitations of the embolic hypothesis. Eur Respir J. 2000;15(3):440-8.

[5] O'Connell C, Montani D, Savale L, Sitbon O, Parent F, Seferian A, et al. Chronic thromboembolic pulmonary hypertension. Presse Médicale. 2015;44(12):e409-16.

[6] Ljungdahl M. es eine Chronische Embolistierung der Lungen Arterie? Dtsch Arch Klin Med. 1928;102:1-23.

[7] Allison PR, Dunnill MS, Marshall R. Pulmonary embolism. Thorax. 1960;15:273-83.

[8] Snyder WA, Kent DC, Baisch BF. Successful endarterectomy of chronically occluded pulmonary artery. Clinical report and physiologic studies. J Thorac Cardiovasc Surg. 1963;45:482-9.

[9] Cabrol C, Cabrol A, Acar J, Gandjbakhch I, Guiraudon G, Laughlin L, et al. Surgical correction of chronic postembolic obstructions of the pulmonary arteries. J Thorac Cardiovasc Surg. 1978;76(5):620-8.

[10] Daily PO, Johnston GG, Simmons CJ, Moser KM. Surgical management of chronic pulmonary embolism: surgical treatment and late results. J Thorac Cardiovasc Surg. 1980;79(4):523-31.

[11] Moser KM, Daily PO, Peterson K, Dembitsky W, Vapnek JM, Shure D, et al. Thromboendarterectomy for chronic, major-vessel thromboembolic pulmonary hypertension. Immediate and long-term results in 42 patients. Ann Intern Med. 1987;107(4):560-5.

[12] Moser KM, Bioor CM. Pulmonary vascular lesions occurring in patients with chronic major vessel thromboembolic pulmonary hypertension. Chest. 1993;103(3):685-92.

[13] Ribeiro A, Lindmarker P, Johnsson H, Juhlin-Dannfelt A, Jorfeldt L. Pulmonary embolism: one-year follow-up with echocardiography Doppler and five-year survival analysis. Circulation. 1999;99(10):1325-30.

[14] Pengo V, Lensing AWA, Prins MH, Marchiori A, Davidson BL, Tiozzo F, et al. Incidence of chronic thromboembolic pulmonary hypertension after pulmonary embolism. N Engl J Med. 2004;350(22):2257-64.

[15] Becattini C, Agnelli G, Pesavento R, Silingardi M, Poggio R, Taliani MR, et al. Incidence of chronic thromboembolic pulmonary hypertension after a first episode of pulmonary embolism. Chest. 2006;130(1):172-5.

[16] Dentali F, Donadini M, Gianni M, Bertolini A, Squizzato A, Venco A, et al. Incidence of chronic pulmonary hypertension in patients with previous pulmonary embolism. Thromb Res. 2009;124(3):256-8.

[17] Lang IM, Madani M. Update on chronic thromboembolic pulmonary hypertension. Circulation. 2014;130(6):508-18.

[18] Wolf M, Boyer-Neumann C, Parent F, Eschwege V, Jaillet H, Meyer D, et al. Thrombotic risk factors in pulmonary hypertension. Eur Respir J. 2000;15(2):395-9.

[19] Morris TA. Why acute pulmonary embolism becomes chronic thromboembolic pulmonary hypertension: clinical and genetic insights. Curr Opin Pulm Med. 2013;19(5):422-429.

[20] Bonderman D, Wilkens H, Wakounig S, Schafers H-J, Jansa P, Lindner J, et al. Risk factors for chronic thromboembolic pulmonary hypertension. Eur Respir J. 2008;33(2):325-31.

[21] Bonderman D, Jakowitsch J, Adlbrecht C, Schemper M, Kyrle PA, Schönauer V, et al. Medical conditions increasing the risk of chronic thromboembolic pulmonary hypertension. Thromb Haemost [Internet]. 2005 [cited 2016 Dec 22]; Available from: http://www.schattauer.de/index.php?id=1214&doi=10.1160/TH04-10-0657&no_cache=1

[22] Bonderman D, Turecek PL, Jakowitsch J, Weltermann A, Adlbrecht C, Schneider B, et al. High prevalence of elevated clotting factor VIII in chronic thromboembolic pulmonary hypertension. Thromb Haemost [Internet]. 2003 [cited 2016 Dec 22]; Available from: http://www.schattauer.de/index.php?id=1214&doi=10.1160/TH03-02-0067&no_cache=1

[23] Jais X. Splenectomy and chronic thromboembolic pulmonary hypertension. Thorax. 2005;60(12):1031-4.

[24] Wynants M, Quarck R, Ronisz A, Alfaro-Moreno E, Van Raemdonck D, Meyns B, et al. Effects of C-reactive protein on human pulmonary vascular cells in chronic thromboembolic pulmonary hypertension. Eur Respir J. 2012;40(4):886-94.

[25] Bonderman D, Jakowitsch J, Redwan B, Bergmeister H, Renner M-K, Panzenbock H, et al. Role for staphylococci in misguided thrombus resolution of chronic thromboembolic pulmonary hypertension. Arterioscler Thromb Vasc Biol. 2008;28(4):678-84.

[26] Nijkeuter M, Hovens MMC, Davidson BL, Huisman MV. Resolution of thromboemboli in patients with acute pulmonary embolism. Chest. 2006;129(1):192-7.

[27] Auger W, Fedullo P. Chronic thromboembolic pulmonary hypertension. Semin Respir Crit Care Med. 2009;30(4):471-83.

[28] Sutton GC, Hall RJ, Kerr IH. Clinical course and late prognosis of treated subacute massive, acute minor, and chronic pulmonary thromboembolism. Heart. 1977;39(10):1135-42.

[29] Riedel M, Stanek V, Widimsky J, Prerovsky I. Longterm follow-up of patients with pulmonary thromboembolism. Chest. 1982;81(2):151-8.

[30] Lewczuk J, Piszko P, Jagas J, Porada A, Sobkowicz B, Wrabec K, et al. Prognostic factors in medically treated patients with chronic pulmonary embolism. Chest. 2001;119(3):818-23.

[31] Chitwood WR, Lyerly HK, Sabiston DC. Surgical management of chronic pulmonary embolism. Ann Surg. 1985;201(1):11-26.

[32] Pepke-Zaba J, Delcroix M, Lang I, Mayer E, Jansa P, Ambroz D, et al. Chronic thromboembolic pulmonary hypertension (CTEPH): results from an international prospective registry. Circulation. 2011;124(18):1973-81.

[33] Dittrich HC, McCann HA, Blanchard DG. Cardiac structure and function in chronic thromboembolic pulmonary hypertension. Am J Card Imag. 1994;8(1):18-27.

[34] Mahmud E, Raisinghani A, Hassankhani A, Sadeghi HM, Strachan GM, Auger W, et al. Correlation of left ventricular diastolic filling characteristics with right ventricular overload and pulmonary artery pressure in chronic thromboembolic pulmonary hypertension. J Am Coll Cardiol. 2002;40(2):318-24.

[35] Tunariu N, Gibbs SJR, Win Z, Gin-Sing W, Graham A, Gishen P, et al. Ventilation-perfusion scintigraphy is more sensitive than multidetector CTPA in detecting chronic thromboembolic pulmonary disease as a treatable cause of pulmonary hypertension. J Nucl Med. 2007;48(5):680-4.

[36] Ryan KL, Fedullo PF, Davis GB, Vasquez TE, Moser KM. Perfusion scan findings understate the severity of angiographic and hemodynamic compromise in chronic thromboembolic pulmonary hypertension. Chest. 1988;93(6):1180-5.

[37] Azarian R, Wartski M, Collignon MA, Parent F, Hervé P, Sors H, et al. Lung perfusion scans and hemodynamics in acute and chronic pulmonary embolism. J Nucl Med Off Publ Soc Nucl Med. 1997;38(6):980-3.

[38] Kerr KM, Auger WR, Fedullo PF, Channick RH, Yi ES, Moser KM. Large vessel pulmonary arteritis mimicking chronic thromboembolic disease. Am J Respir Crit Care Med. 1995;152(1):367-73.

[39] Bailey CL, Channick RN, Auger WR, Fedullo PF, Kerr KM, Yung GL, et al. "High probability" perfusion lung scans in pulmonary venoocclusive disease. Am J Respir Crit Care Med. 2000;162(5):1974-8.

[40] Kauczor HU, Schwickert HC, Mayer E, Kersjes W, Moll R, Schweden F. Pulmonary artery sarcoma mimicking chronic thromboembolic disease: computed tomography and magnetic resonance imaging findings. Cardiovasc Intervent Radiol. 1994;17(4):185-9.

[41] Bergin CJ, Rios G, King MA, Belezzuoli E, Luna J, Auger WR. Accuracy of high-resolution CT in identifying chronic pulmonary thromboembolic disease. Am J Roentgenol. 1996;166(6):1371-7.

[42] Gefter WB, Hatabu H, Holland GA, Gupta KB, Henschke CI, Palevsky HI. Pulmonary thromboembolism: recent developments in diagnosis with CT and MR imaging. Radiology. 1995;197(3):561-74.

[43] Perlmutt LM, Braun SD, Newman GE, Oke EJ, Dunnick NR. Pulmonary arteriography in the high-risk patient. Radiology. 1987;162(1):187-9.

[44] Auger WR, Fedullo PF, Moser KM, Buchbinder M, Peterson KL. Chronic major-vessel thromboembolic pulmonary artery obstruction: appearance at angiography. Radiology. 1992;182(2):393-8.

[45] Surie S, Gibson NS, Gerdes VEA, Bouma BJ, van Eck – Smit BLF, Buller HR, et al. Active search for chronic thromboembolic pulmonary hypertension does not appear indicated after acute pulmonary embolism. Thromb Res. 2010;125(5):e202-5.

[46] Galiè N, Humbert M, Vachiery J-L, Gibbs S, Lang I, Torbicki A, et al. ESC/ERS guidelines for the diagnosis and treatment of pulmonary hypertension: the joint task force for the diagnosis and treatment of pulmonary hypertension of the European Society of Cardiology (ESC) and the European Respiratory Society (ERS) endorsed by: Association for European Paediatric and Congenital Cardiology (AEPC), International Society for Heart and Lung Transplantation (ISHLT). Eur Respir J. 2015;46(4):903-75.

[47] Authors/Task Force Members, Torbicki A, Perrier A, Konstantinides S, Agnelli G, Galie N, et al. Guidelines on the diagnosis and management of acute pulmonary embolism: the task force for the diagnosis and management of acute pulmonary embolism of the European Society of Cardiology (ESC). Eur Heart J. 2008;29(18):2276-315.

[48] Klok FA, Surie S, Kempf T, Eikenboom J, van Straalen JP, van Kralingen KW, et al. A simple non-invasive diagnostic algorithm for ruling out chronic thromboembolic pulmonary hypertension in patients after acute pulmonary embolism. Thromb Res. 2011;128(1):21-6.

[49] Shure D, Gregoratos G, Moser KM. Fiberoptic angioscopy: role in the diagnosis of chronic pulmonary arterial obstruction. Ann Intern Med. 1985;103(6 (Pt 1)):844-50.

[50] Keogh AM, Mayer E, Benza RL, Corris P, Dartevelle PG, Frost AE, et al. Interventional and surgical modalities of treatment in pulmonary hypertension. J Am Coll Cardiol. 2009;54(1):S67-77.

[51] Jenkins DP, Madani M, Mayer E, Kerr K, Kim N, Klepetko W, et al. Surgical treatment of chronic thromboembolic pulmonary hypertension. Eur Respir J. 2013;41(3):735-42.

[52] Fedullo PF, Auger WR, Kerr KM, Rubin LJ. Chronic thromboembolic pulmonary hypertension. N Engl J Med. 2001;345(20):1465-72.

[53] Jamieson SW, Kapelanski DP, Sakakibara N, Manecke GR, Thistlethwaite PA, Kerr KM, et al. Pulmonary endarterectomy: experience and lessons learned in 1500 cases. Ann Thorac Surg. 2003;76(5):1457-64.

[54] Masuda M, Nakajima N. Our experience of surgical treatment for chronic pulmonary thromboembolism. Ann Thorac Cardiovasc Surg Off J Assoc Thorac Cardiovasc Surg Asia. 2001;7(5):261-5.

[55] Mayer E, Kramm T, Dahm M, Moersig W, Eberle B, Düber C, et al. Early results of pulmonary thromboendarterectomy in chronic thromboembolic pulmonary hypertension. Z Kardiol. 1997;86(11):920-7.

[56] Gilbert TB, Gaine SP, Rubin LJ, Sequeira AJ. Short-term outcome and predictors of adverse events following pulmonary thromboendarterectomy. World J Surg. 1998;22(10):1029-32; discussion 1033.

[57] Rubens FD, Bourke M, Hynes M, Nicholson D, Kotrec M, Boodhwani M, et al. Surgery for chronic thromboembolic pulmonary hypertension—inclusive experience from a National Referral Center. Ann Thorac Surg. 2007;83(3):1075-81.

[58] Mellemkjær S, Ilkjær LB, Klaaborg KE, Christiansen CL, Severinsen IK, Nielsen-Kudsk JE, et al. Pulmonary endarterectomy for chronic thromboembolic pulmonary hypertension. Ten years experience in Denmark. Scand Cardiovasc J. 2006;40(1):49-53.

[59] Madani MM, Jamieson SW. Technical advances of pulmonary endarterectomy for chronic thromboembolic pulmonary hypertension. Semin Thorac Cardiovasc Surg. 2006;18(3):243-9.

[60] Kouchoukos NBE, Hanley FKJ. Chronic pulmonary thromboembolic disease. In: Cardiac surgery, 4th ed. Philadelphia: Elsevier, Saunders; 2013, pp. 1028-34.

[61] Jamieson SW, Auger WR, Fedullo PF, Channick RN, Kriett JM, Tarazi RY, et al. Experience and results with 150 pulmonary thromboendarterectomy operations over a 29-month period. J Thorac Cardiovasc Surg. 1993;106(1):116-26; discussion 126-7.

[62] Thistlethwaite PA, Auger WR, Madani MM, Pradhan S, Kapelanski DP, Jamieson SW. Pulmonary thromboendarterectomy combined with other cardiac operations: indications, surgical approach, and outcome. Ann Thorac Surg. 2001;72(1):13-8.

[63] Kerr KM, Auger WR, Marsh JJ, Comito RM, Fedullo RL, Smits GJ, et al. The use of cylexin (CY-1503) in prevention of reperfusion lung injury in patients undergoing pulmonary thromboendarterectomy. Am J Respir Crit Care Med. 2000;162(1):14-20.

[64] Jamieson SW, Kapelanski DP. Pulmonary endarterectomy. Curr Probl Surg. 2000;37(3):165-252.

[65] D'Armini A. Pulmonary thromboendarterectomy in patients with chronic thromboembolic pulmonary hypertension: hemodynamic characteristics and changes. Eur J Cardiothorac Surg. 2000;18(6):696-702.

[66] Mares P, Gilbert TB, Tschernko EM, Hiesmayr M, Muhm M, Herneth A, et al. Pulmonary artery thromboendarterectomy: a comparison of two different postoperative treatment strategies: Anesth Analg. 2000;90(2):267.

[67] Rubens F, Wells P, Bencze S, Bourke M. Surgical treatment of chronic thromboembolic pulmonary hypertension. Can Respir J. 2000;7(1):49-57.

[68] Saouti N, Morshuis WJ, Heijmen RH, Snijder RJ. Long-term outcome after pulmonary endarterectomy for chronic thromboembolic pulmonary hypertension: a single institution experience. Eur J Cardiothorac Surg. 2009;35(6):947-52.

[69] Archibald CJ, Auger WR, Fedullo PF, Channick RN, Kerr KM, Jamieson SW, et al. Long-term outcome after pulmonary thromboendarterectomy. Am J Respir Crit Care Med. 1999;160(2):523-8.

[70] Mayer E, Dahm M, Hake U, Schmid FX, Pitton M, Kupferwasser I, et al. Mid-term results of pulmonary thromboendarterectomy for chronic thromboembolic pulmonary hypertension. Ann Thorac Surg. 1996;61(6):1788-92.

[71] Hartz RS, Byrne JG, Levitsky S, Park J, Rich S. Predictors of mortality in pulmonary thromboendarterectomy. Ann Thorac Surg. 1996;62(5):1255-60.

[72] Miller WT, Osiason AW, Langlotz CP, Palevsky HI. Reperfusion edema after thromboendarterectomy: radiographic patterns of disease. J Thorac Imag. 1998;13(3):178-83.

[73] Dartevelle P. Angioscopic video-assisted pulmonary endarterectomy for post-embolic pulmonary hypertension. Eur J Cardiothorac Surg. 1999;16(1):38-43.

[74] Ando M, Okita Y, Tagusari O, Kitamura S, Nakanishi N, Kyotani S. Surgical treatment for chronic thromboembolic pulmonary hypertension under profound hypothermia and circulatory arrest in 24 patients. J Card Surg. 1999;14(5):377-85.

[75] Corsico AG, D'Armini AM, Cerveri I, Klersy C, Ansaldo E, Niniano R, et al. Long-term outcome after pulmonary endarterectomy. Am J Respir Crit Care Med. 2008;178(4):419-24.

[76] Mo M, Kapelanski DP, Mitruka SN, Auger WR, Fedullo PF, Channick RN, et al. Reoperative pulmonary thromboendarterectomy. Ann Thorac Surg. 1999;68(5):1770-6.

Chapter 4

Pulmonary Embolism

Fayaz Ahmed and Ahmed Elsayed Mahmoud

Additional information is available at the end of the chapter

http://dx.doi.org/10.5772/68040

Abstract

Pulmonary embolism is sudden occlusion of pulmonary arteries, usually by a clot arising in the lower limb veins. The majority of pulmonary emboli are silent, and it is only when the embolus burden is substantial that the patient becomes symptomatic. Mortality after an acute, major thromboembolic episode is significantly high. Pulmonary embolism which causes hemodynamic instability is usually associated with occlusion of more than 50% of the pulmonary vasculature. Associated severe pulmonary hypertension may cause cardiac arrest. The precipitation of RV failure is also affected by the degree of preexisting right ventricular hypertrophy or dilatation, tricuspid valve regurgitation, and the presence of coronary artery disease. Aggressive therapy is needed in this subgroup of patients. Unfortunately, surgical embolectomy is seldom even entertained as an option in the management of these patients. A critical assessment of the data reveals that there is in fact a definite place for surgical therapy in the management of massive pulmonary embolism.

Keywords: pulmonary embolism, pulmonary hypertension, surgical embolectomy

1. Introduction

Pulmonary embolism is sudden occlusion of pulmonary arteries, usually by a clot arising in the lower limb veins. It is not a disease by itself but rather a complication of this venous thrombosis.

Pulmonary embolism is commonly mislabeled, more likely an unrecognized phenomenon particularly in hospitalized individuals.

The majority of pulmonary emboli are silent, and it is only when the embolus burden is substantial that the patient becomes symptomatic. Mortality after an acute, major thromboembolic episode reaches about 15–20% of patients within 48 hours [1].

Aggressive therapy is needed in this subgroup of patients. Unfortunately, surgical embolectomy is seldom even entertained as an option in the management of these patients, published mortality rates for acute pulmonary embolectomy have ranged from 20 to 60%, making it difficult to argue that the surgical results were any better than the natural history. A critical assessment of the data reveals that there is in fact a definite place for surgical therapy in the management of massive pulmonary embolism [2].

2. Practice essentials

Pulmonary embolism usually presents with dyspnea, tachypnea, dull chest pain, and cardiovascular changes such as tachycardia, mild-to-moderate hypotension, and distended neck veins. Most pulmonary embolism patients are hemodynamically stable and have adequate cardiac output.

Pulmonary embolism which causes hemodynamic instability is termed massive pulmonary embolism. It is usually associated with occlusion of more than 50% of the pulmonary vasculature [3]. Pulmonary angiograms demonstrate a unique degree of blockage of the pulmonary vasculature.

The severity of symptoms may not be related to the embolus burden, particularly in patients with preexisting cardiac or pulmonary disease. Cardiac arrest may occur. The precipitation of RV failure is also affected by the degree of right ventricular hypertrophy or dilatation, tricuspid valve regurgitation, and the presence of coronary artery disease. Pulmonary hypertension is also influenced by many factors. Humoral factors such as serotonin, adenosine diphosphate (ADP), platelet-derived growth factor (PDGF), and thromboxane are released from platelets attached to the thrombi. Anoxia and tissue ischemia downstream from emboli inhibit endothelium-derived relaxing factor (EDRF) production and enhance release of superoxide anions by activated neutrophils [4].

2.1. Anatomy

The anatomy of the pulmonary vasculature should be familiar to all cardiothoracic surgeons. What may be less well appreciated, however, is the remarkable access available to the lobar vessels via median sternotomy. All lobar and segmental vessels can be accessed via incisions in the pulmonary arteries from within the pericardial space as one would during pulmonary thrombo-endarterectomy [5].

2.2. Pathophysiology

Pathophysiology of pulmonary hypertension in acute pulmonary embolism entails the release of serotonin from platelets, histamine from tissues, and circulating thrombin. Hypoxia due to ventilation/perfusion mismatch and increased dead space will also worsen pulmonary vasoconstriction and set a vicious cycle. Persistent systemic hypotension or refractory hypoxemia is an indication for aggressive interventional, surgical, or thrombolytic management. Operative risk is markedly elevated once the patient is in cardiogenic shock [6].

http://dx.doi.org/10.5772/68040

Right ventricular dysfunction is a harbinger of hemodynamic decompensation, an event that may unfold quite precipitously, abruptly closing the window of opportunity on a patient that has been otherwise holding on for several hours. Thrombolytics have taken center stage in the aggressive treatment of the unstable patient [7]. This is in part due to their wide availability and the familiarity many physicians have with their use in the context of treating acute coronary syndromes. However, study reports found no improvement in mortality rate when thrombolytics were used in unselected patients as compared with heparin but an almost two-fold increased risk of hemorrhage. Catheter embolectomy is another option. Endovascular techniques include clot fragmentation, clot aspiration, and rheolytic therapy. The mortality rate associated with these interventions, however, has been 25–30% [8]. Surgical intervention performed before hemodynamic collapse has an operative risk no higher than that of thrombolytic therapy in most cases. Surgery is clearly the option of choice when there is a clot in transit, in the right atrium, or trapped in a patent foramen ovale [7, 9].

3. Diagnosis

Diagnosis is suspected with a history consistent with massive pulmonary embolism. Symptoms and signs vary with the extent of blockage, the magnitude of humoral response, and the cardiac and pulmonary reserve of the patient. Routine laboratory tests are usually normal. Serum D-dimer is almost always elevated in the presence of acute pulmonary embolus and is frequently used in emergency rooms as a screening test. The most common electrocardiographic abnormalities of acute pulmonary embolism are tachycardia and nonspecific ST- and T-wave changes [5]. The major value of the electrocardiogram is excluding a myocardial infarction. A minority of patients with massive embolism may show evidence of corpulmonale, right axis deviation, or right bundle branch block. Chest X-ray may show oligemia (Westermark's sign) or linear atelectasis (Fleischner lines), both of which are nonspecific findings. Ventilation-perfusion (V/Q) scans may be used for their negative predictive value and may be unreliable because of pneumonia, atelectasis, previous pulmonary emboli, and other conditions may cause a ventilation and perfusion mismatch. In general, negative V/Q scan may rule out significant pulmonary embolism. Pulmonary angiogram provides the most definitive diagnosis for acute pulmonary embolism. Contrast-enhanced high-resolution computerized tomographic (CT) scanning is most commonly diagnostic (**Figure 1**).

Advantages of MDCTPA in the diagnosis of acute PE are as follows:

- Widely available, especially after day hours
- Rapid interpretation
- Direct visualization of embolus
- Noninvasive
- Highly accurate
- Evaluation of alternative causes of chest pain
- Possible concurrent performance of lower extremity

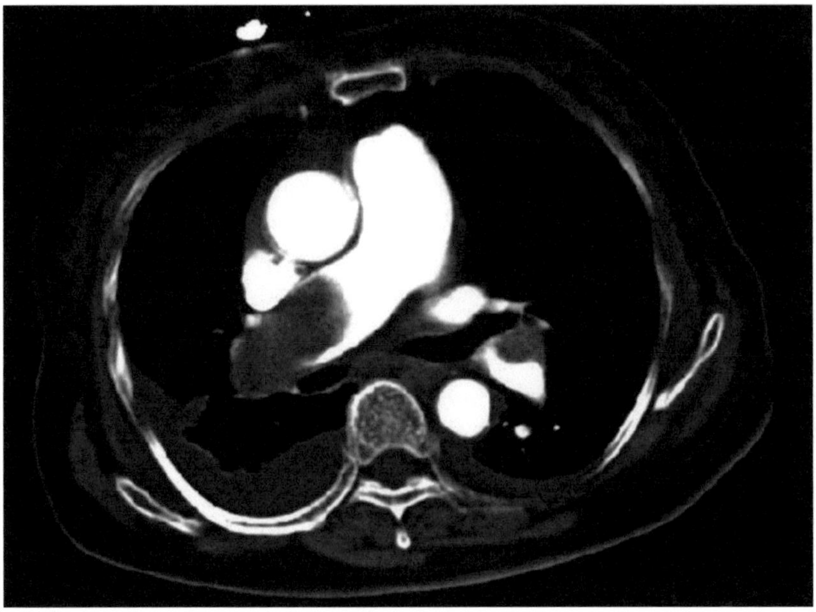

Figure 1. Massive PE as appears in contrast enhanced CT chest.

- venous imaging with CTV
- Ability to provide ancillary findings, which may affect management and prognosis [CTV (computed tomographic venography) and MDCTPA (multidetector computed tomographic pulmonary angiography)].

The most important recent diagnostic development from a surgical standpoint is transesophageal echocardiography. This modality may not visualize distal embolic material in the pulmonary vasculature but is more important to identify thrombus in transit, including paradoxical embolus in transit, and to permit evaluation of right ventricular function (**Figure 2**) [10].

4. Treatment

Oxygen should be administered to alleviate hypoxic pulmonary vasoconstriction, and it is likely that a severely affected patient will require intubation and ventilator support. Pharmacological agents, including vasopressors, may be instituted to stabilize the patient.

Pulmonary artery catheters, although obviously helpful in management, may occasionally emboli more thrombi because of the risk of dislodging further thromboembolic material [11].

4.1. Thrombolysis

Natural history of the clot in survivors of acute embolic events is fragmentation and progressive lysis. Thrombolytic agents dissolve thrombi by activating plasminogen to plasmin.

http://dx.doi.org/10.5772/68040

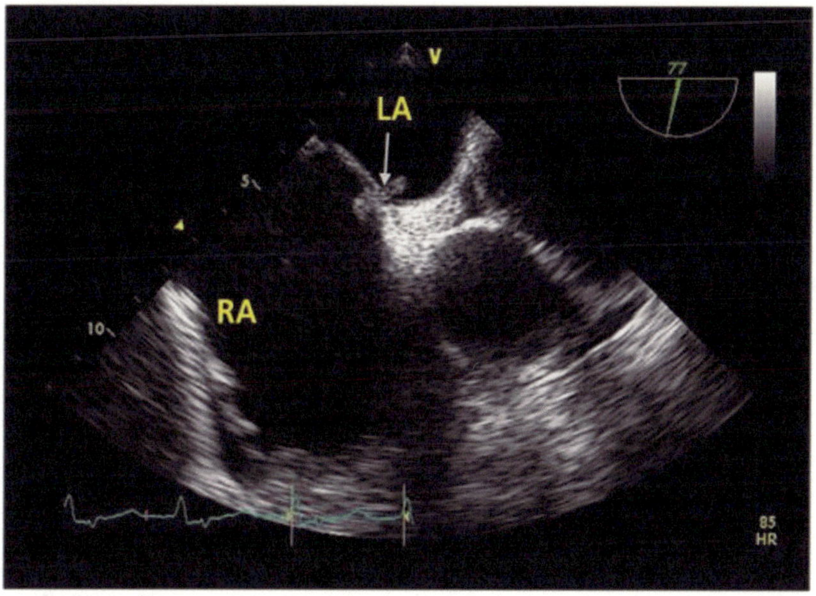

Figure 2. Echocardiogram demonstrating thrombus in transit across PFO.

Plasmin, when in proximity to a thrombus, degrades fibrin to soluble peptides. Circulating plasmin also degrades soluble fibrinogen and, to variable degrees, factors II, V, and VIII. In addition, increased concentrations of fibrin and fibrinogen degradation products contribute to coagulopathy by both inhibiting the conversion of fibrinogen to fibrin and interfering with fibrin polymerization. The thrombolytic agents currently reported for the treatment of acute pulmonary embolism include streptokinase, urokinase, recombinant tissue plasminogen activator (rt-PA, alteplase), anisoylated plasminogen streptokinase activator complex (APSAC, anistreplase), and reteplase [12]. There are newer agents arriving, like tenecteplase, lanoteplase, staphylokinase, and saruplase and are undergoing clinical testing.

Trials suggest a trend toward better results with thrombolytic therapy because of a more rapid diminution in right ventricular afterload and dysfunction. Compared with heparin therapy alone, thrombolytic agents carry a higher risk of bleeding problems, with up to 20% of patients experiencing a significant bleeding complication [13]. In general, thrombolytic therapy is contraindicated in patients with fresh surgical wounds, anemia, recent stroke, peptic ulcer, or bleeding dyscrasias.

4.2. Anticoagulation

Patients should be heparinized to prevent further propagation of thrombus at its origin and also in the pulmonary arterial tree. Intravenous (IV) heparin is started with an initial bolus dose of 70 U/kg followed by 18–20 U/kg/h. Heparin prevents propagation and formation of new thrombus. It rarely dissolves existing clot. Intrinsic fibrinolytic system will lyse fresh thrombi over a period of days to weeks. Evidence suggests early treatment of stable patients with acute pulmonary embolism with subcutaneous low-molecular-weight heparin (tinzaparin) given once daily has been shown to be as effective and safe as IV heparin with respect to recurrent thromboembolism, major bleeding, and death [14].

4.3. Surgical embolectomy

Emergency pulmonary embolectomy was first described by Trendelenburg in 1908, using pulmonary artery and aortic occlusion, through a transthoracic approach. There were no surviving patients [14]. Later on, the first successful open embolectomy was performed and described by Sharp using cardiopulmonary bypass [15].

If a patient has been taken directly to the operating room without a definitive diagnosis, transesophageal or epicardial echocardiography and color Doppler mapping can confirm or refute the diagnosis in the operating room.

4.3.1. Indication for surgery

Emergency pulmonary thromboembolectomy is indicated for suitable patients with life-threatening circulatory insufficiency, where the diagnosis of acute pulmonary embolism has been established. Indications for acute surgical intervention include the following: hemodynamic instability, definitive diagnosis of pulmonary embolism in the main or lobar pulmonary arteries with compromise of gas exchange, unstable patients in whom thrombolytic or anticoagulation therapy is absolutely contraindicated, thrombus in transit or thrombus trapped within the right atrium, patent foramen ovale, or right ventricle.

Surgical embolectomy, as initial therapy for massive PE compared to thrombolytic therapy, has less early mortality rates and significantly less bleeding complications.

Patients who undergo surgical embolectomy after the failure of lysis clearly demonstrate a critically high-mortality rate.

CT-derived RV/LV ratio could be a useful parameter to identify candidates who might benefit from direct surgical therapy instead of thrombolysis [16].

4.3.2. Operative procedure

Intraoperative transesophageal echocardiography is now a routine in modern practice and greatly facilitates intraoperative decision-making particularly with regard to exploration of the right atrium and evaluation for clot in transit [10]. The groin vessels should be prepped into the field in case postoperative extracorporeal membrane oxygenation is necessary. Poor venous return from the inferior vena cava line only can be a result of clot in transit impacted in the cannula orifice (**Figure 3**). For this reason, the superior vena cava cannula is placed first so that partial bypass may be initiated if clot is dislodged from the inferior vena cava. Routine massage of the lower extremities and abdomen and open aspiration of the inferior vena cava return with cardiotomy suckers is better to extract additional material in transit. Tapes are passed around the superior vena cava and inferior vena cava, if patent foramen ovale or paradoxic embolus in transit has been identified by transesophageal echo. A brief episode of cardioplegic arrest should be instituted to examine the left atrium (**Figure 4**).

http://dx.doi.org/10.5772/68040

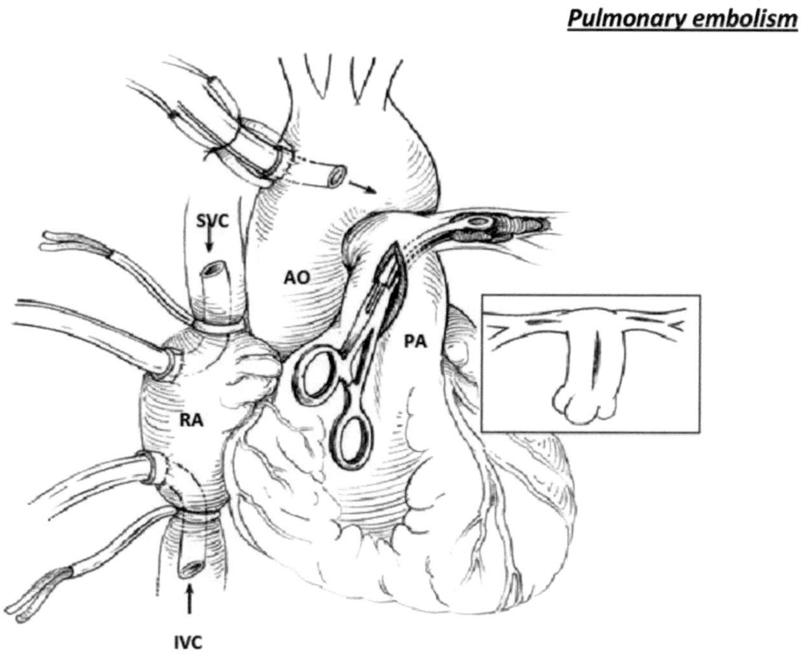

Figure 3. The pulmonary arteriotomy sites.

If embolus in transit is identified in the right atrium, this can be extracted via a standard right atrial incision without cardioplegic arrest (**Figure 4**). This approach provides optimal protection of the right ventricle during the procedure. If right atrial exploration is not required,

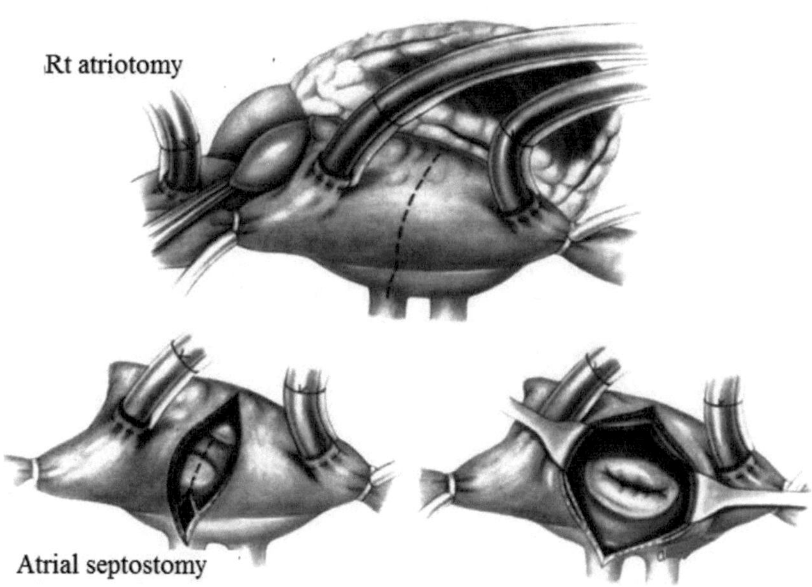

Figure 4. Approaches to explore thrombus in transit.

a bullet-tip sucker can be dropped into the right atrium via a stab wound with a purse-string suture. This will reduce the amount of blood passing through the right ventricle and into the pulmonary artery [11, 17].

The pulmonary vessels are extraordinarily fragile and rapidly taper in diameter, making rupture of the vessels a very real possibility. Thrombus in the left pulmonary artery is accessed via an incision beginning in the main pulmonary artery. Adequate access permitting direct visualization of the segmental vessels requires extension of the incision onto the left pulmonary artery itself. This may require division of the pericardial reflection over the ventral surface of the pulmonary artery (**Figure 5**).

A linear incision first in the posterior pericardium overlying the vessel and then in the vessel itself provides ready access to all of the lobar and segmental vessels. An incision such as this permits direct inspection of the right upper lobe branch, right middle lobe branch, and the segmental vessels to the right lower lobe. A flexible suction catheter passed in the pulmonary arteries with massage of the lungs, helps to dislodge smaller thrombi in the distal branches (**Figure 6**). The arteriotomies are primarily closed with running 4-0 Prolene. A final step in the procedure is insertion of an inferior vena cava filter via a purse-string suture on the right atrial appendage.

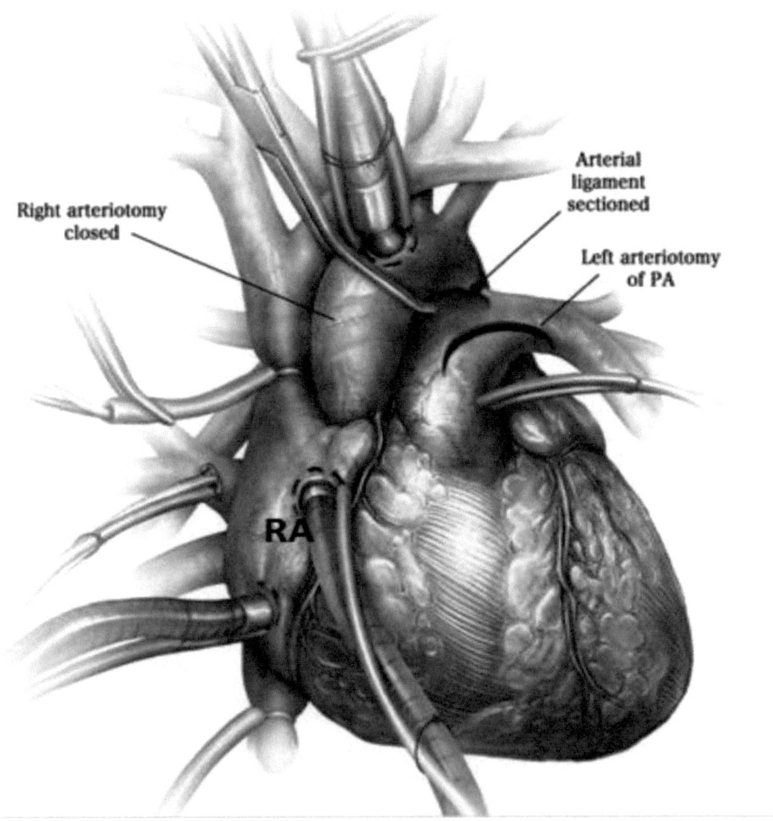

Figure 5. Incision to explore distal pulmonary arteries.

http://dx.doi.org/10.5772/68040

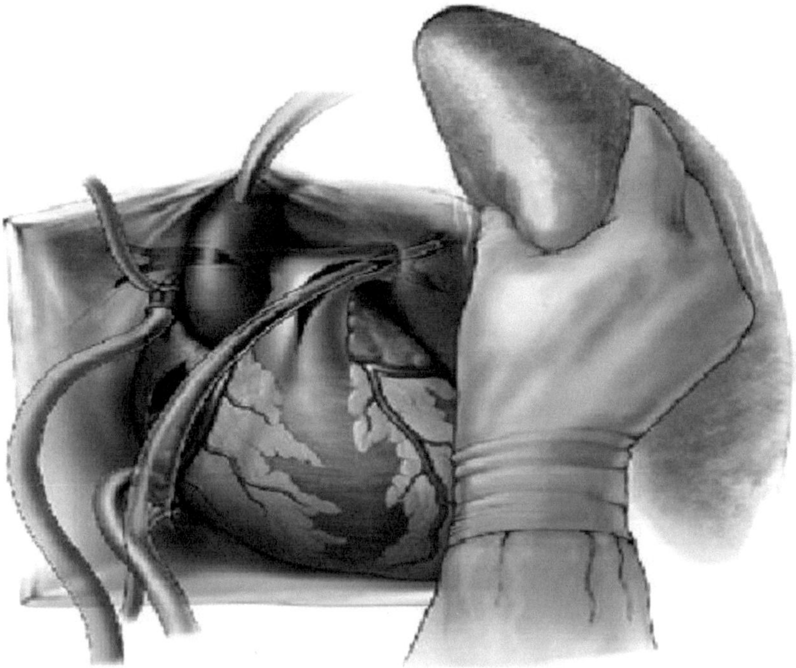

Figure 6. Lung massage to mobilise peripheral thrombi.

4.3.3. Benefits of surgery

Pulmonary embolectomies demonstrate excellent early and late survival rates for patients with stable PE and unstable PE. These findings confirm pulmonary embolectomy as a beneficial therapeutic option for central PE, especially during the postoperative period when thrombolytic therapy is often contraindicated. Procoagulant risk factors such as endothelial injury, malignancy, and decreased mobility are common among postoperative patient populations across surgical specialties, but surgical options for the treatment of PE remain underappreciated and underutilized. With increasing surgical experience and improved outcomes, the role for pulmonary embolectomy in the acute setting may be expanding [18, 19]. All PE patients with imminent risk of hemodynamic decompensation due to severe RV impairment and central clot burden should be evaluated for surgical treatment [20]. Surgical embolectomy although normally confined to the most critical PE patients can be done with good long-term survival comparable to active medical treatment with thrombolysis despite the mortality risk inflicted by the surgical procedure. High-risk PE patients treated with surgical embolectomy had a significantly lower amount of residual emboli and pulmonary diffusion impairment than patients treated with thrombolysis. The clinical consequences of residual emboli were identified significant shorter 6-MWT, a higher mean pulmonary arterial pressure, and more dyspnea when compared to PE patients without residual emboli [21]. Residual clot burden is an independent risk factor for increased mortality at long-term follow-up [22]. Residual emboli after acute PE were found to be an independent predictor for chronic thromboembolic pulmonary hypertension, a severe late complication of acute PE [21, 22].

Pulmonary diffusion impairment after acute PE occurs more frequently in high-risk patients treated with thrombolysis compared to surgical embolectomy and was correlated with residual emboli. The surgical superiority on pulmonary morbidity is due to rapid removal of the total emboli resulting in fast restoration of normal pulmonary circulation, while thrombolysis either is unable to resolve the emboli due to its size or fractionates it into smaller parts which are carried to the peripheral pulmonary vasculature.

Current American Heart Association, European Society of Cardiology, and American College of Chest Physicians guidelines reserve surgical pulmonary embolectomy for central PE with hemodynamic instability and a contraindication for thrombolytic therapy, or when thrombolysis has failed [23, 24]. These treatment algorithms are based on limited data from small surgical series, and these practice patterns may be more reflective of scarce surgical expertise. Increasing evidence suggests that pulmonary embolectomy might be considered first-line therapy for select patients [25, 26]. This has resulted in the extension of eligibility for pulmonary embolectomy to include those who are hemodynamically stable but with demonstrative evidence of impending right ventricular failure [27].

5. ECMO in pulmonary embolism

Extracorporeal membrane oxygenation use (ECMO) for selected patients with massive PE is associated with good outcomes. Patients presenting in cardiac arrest have worse outcomes. Survival rates and neurological recovery are better when the cause of cardiac arrest is pulmonary embolism compared to other causes of cardiac arrest [11].

As an emergency procedure, standard femoro-femoral, venoarterial ECMO is instituted to ensure rapid and effective CPR in arrest or pre arrest patients, this can be achieved by use of smaller percutaneous cannulas limited to basic one arterial and one venous cannula (**Figure 7**) [5].

The tip of the venous catheter is advanced into the right atrium to obtain a flow rate of 2.5–4.0 l/min using an emergency pump-oxygenator circuit primed with crystalloid.

Mortality rates for emergency pulmonary thromboembolectomy vary widely between 11 and 92% in retrospective studies with varying operative techniques, preoperative hemodynamic state of the patient populations, and treatment plans. In general, greater surgical mortality was encountered if a patient had a preoperative cardiac arrest or required ECMO support [9, 28].

Prevention of recurrence should always be stressed upon in patients with successful outcomes, by addressing factors such as obesity, tobacco abuse, use of oral contraceptives, or postmenopausal hormone replacement. Consideration should be given to a search for occult malignancy. Consultation with a hematologist and systematic search for a prothrombotic state is routine. If no treatable cause is identifiable or patients have evidence of a hypercoagulable state, warfarin therapy is indicated for life.

http://dx.doi.org/10.5772/68040

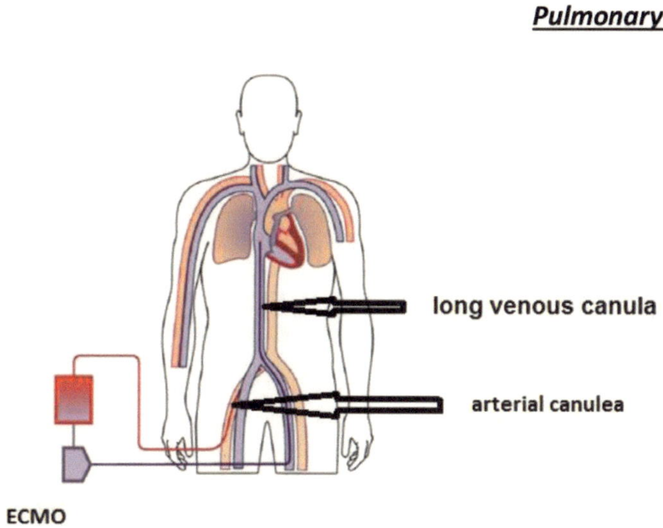

Figure 7. Arteriovenous ECMO circuit.

Author details

Fayaz Ahmed* and Ahmed Elsayed Mahmoud

*Address all correspondence to: drfayaz@gmail.com

King Fahd Hospital of the University, AlKhobar, Saudi Arabia

References

[1] Wakefield TW, Proctor MC. Current status of pulmonary embolism and venous thrombosis prophylaxis. Seminars in Vascular Surgery. 2000;**13**:171–181

[2] Goldhaber SZ, Visani L, De Rosa M. Acute pulmonary embolism: Clinical outcomes in the International Cooperative Pulmonary Embolism Registry [ICOPER]. Lancet. 1999;**353**:1386

[3] Hoagland PM. Massive Pulmonary Embolism. In. Goldhaber SZ, Pulmonary Embolism and Deep Vein Thrombosis, Philadelphia: W.B. Saunders; 1986. p. 179

[4] Gurewich V, Cohen ML, Thomas DP. Humoral factors in massive pulmonary embolism: An experimental study. American Heart Journal. 1968;**76**:784–794

[5] Goldhaber SZ, Elliott CG. Acute pulmonary embolism: Part I: Epidemiology, pathophysiology, and diagnosis. Circulation. 2003;**108**(22):2726

[6] Spagnoloa S, Barbatoa L, Grassob M A, Tesler UF. Retrograde pulmonary perfusion as an adjunct to standard pulmonary embolectomy for acute pulmonary embolism. Multimedia Manual of Cardiothoracic Surgery. 2014; pii: mmu019. doi:10.1093/mmcts/mmu019

[7] Cho Y H, Sung K, Kim WS, SeopJeong AD, Lee YT, Park PW, Kim DK. Management of acute massive pulmonary embolism: Is surgical embolectomy inferior to thrombolysis? International Journal of Cardiology. 2016;**203**:579–583

[8] Greenfield LJ, Proctor MC, Williams DM, et al. Long-term experience with transvenous catheter pulmonary embolectomy. Journal of Vascular Surgery. 1993;**18**:450–458

[9] Lehnert P, Møller CH, Mortensen J, Kjaergaard J, Olsen PS, Carlsen J. Surgical embolectomy compared to thrombolysis in acute pulmonary embolism: Morbidity and mortality. European Journal of Cardiothoracic Surgery 2016; doi:10.1093/ejcts/ezw297.

[10] Yalamanchili K, Fleisher AG, Lehrman SG, Axelrod HI, Lafaro RJ, Sarabu MR, Zias EA, Moggio RA. Open pulmonary embolectomy for treatment of major pulmonary embolism. Annals of Thoracic Surgery. 2004;**77**:819–823

[11] Goldhaber SZ, Elliott CG. Acute pulmonary embolism: Part II: Risk stratification, treatment, and prevention. Circulation 2003;**108**:2834

[12] Riedel M. Therapy for pulmonary thromboembolism. Part 1: Acute massive pulmonary embolism. Cor Vasa. 1996;**38**:93–102

[13] Heiberg J, Lars B. Ilkjær: Pulmonary endarterectomy after pulmonary infectious embolisms. Interactive CardioVascular and Thoracic Surgery. 2013;**16**:556–557. doi:10.1093/icvts/ivs523 Advance Access publication 17 December 2012

[14] Dalen JE, Banas Jr JS, Brooks HL, et al. Resolution rate of pulmonary embolism in man. New England Journal of Medicine. 1969;**280**:1194–1199

[15] Sharp EH. Pulmonary embolectomy: Successful removal of a massive pulmonary embolus with the support of cardiopulmonary bypass—a case report. Annals of Surgery. 1962;**156**:1–4

[16] Aymarda T, Kadnera A, Widmera A, Bascianib R, Tevaearaia H, Webera A, Schmidlia J, Carrela T. Massive pulmonary embolism: Surgical embolectomy versus thrombolytic therapy—should surgical indications be revisited? European Journal of Cardiothoracic Surgery. 2013;**43**:90–94. doi:10.1093/ejcts/ezs123 Advance Access publication 30 March 2012.

[17] Jakob H, Vahl C, Lange R, et al. Modified surgical concept for fulminant pulmonary embolism. European J ournal of Cardiothoracic Surgery. 1995;**9**:557

[18] Konstantinides SV, Torbicki A, Agnelli G, et al. 2014 ESC Guidelines on the diagnosis and management of acute pulmonary embolism: The task force for the diagnosis and management of acute pulmonary embolism of the European Society of Cardiology (ESC). European Heart Journal. 2014;**29**:2276–315

[19] Goldhaber SZ. Surgical pulmonary embolectomy: The resurrection of an almost discarded operation. Texas Heart Institute Journal. 2013;**40**:5–8

[20] Stein PD, Alnas M, Beemath A, et al. Outcome of pulmonary embolectomy. American Journal of Cardiology. 2007;**99**:421–423

[21] Samoukovic G, Malas T, deVarennes B. The role of pulmonary embolectomy in the treatment of acute pulmonary embolism: A literature review from 1968 to 2008. Interactive Cardiovascular and Thoracic Surgery. 2010;**11**:265–70

[22] Meyer G, Vicaut E, Danays T, et al. Fibrinolysis for patients with intermediate-risk pulmonary embolism. New England Journal of Medicine. 2014;**370**:1402–11

[23] Jaff MR, McMurtry MS, Archer SL, et al. American Heart Association Council on Cardiopulmonary, Critical Care, Perioperative and Resuscitation, American Heart Association Council on Peripheral Vascular Disease, American Heart Association Council on Arteriosclerosis, Thrombosis and Vascular Biology. Management of massive and submassive pulmonary embolism, iliofemoral deep vein thrombosis, andchronic thromboembolic pulmonary hypertension: A scientific statement from the American Heart Association. Circulation. 2011;**123**:1788–1830

[24] Kearon C, Akl EA, Comerota AJ, et al. Antithrombotic therapyfor VTE disease: Antithrombotic therapy and preventionof thrombosis, 9th ed: American College of Chest Physiciansevidence-based clinical practice guidelines. Chest. 2012;**141**(Suppl):e419–494.

[25] Leacche M, Unic D, Goldhaber SZ, et al. Modern surgicaltreatment of massive pulmonary embolism: Results in 47consecutive patients after rapid diagnosis and aggressivesurgical approach. Journal of Thoracic and Cardiovascular Surgery. 2005;**12**:1018–1023

[26] Amirghofran AA, Nia AE, Javan R, et al. Surgical embolectomyin acute massive pulmonary embolism. Asian Cardiovascular and Thoracic Annals. 2007;**15**:149–153

[27] Neely RC, Byrne JG, Gosev I, Cohn LH, Javed Q, Rawn JD, Goldhaber SZ, Piazza G, Aranki SF, Shekar PS, Leacche M. Surgical embolectomy for acute massive and submassive pulmonary embolism in a series of 115 Patients. Annals of Thoracic Surgery. 2015; **100**:1245–52

[28] Yusuff HO, Zochios V, Vuylsteke A. Extracorporeal membrane oxygenation in acute massive pulmonary embolism: A systematic review, sagepub.co.uk/journalsPermissions.nav doi: 10.1177/0267659115583377, prf.sagepub.com.

Chapter 5

Thromboembolism in Renal Diseases

Milena Nikolova-Vlahova, Marta Petrova Baleva and Petar Krasimirov Nikolov

Additional information is available at the end of the chapter

http://dx.doi.org/10.5772/intechopen.68486

Abstract

Patients with renal diseases are prone to both thrombosis and bleeding, as they have profound changes in all three classic components of coagulation, defined approximately 150 years ago by Virchow: blood flow, vessel wall (endothelial injury), and coagulation properties of the blood (e.g., coagulation and fibrinolytic systems and platelets). The prothrombotic state in chronic kidney disease (CKD), glomerular diseases (including systemic lupus and vasculitis), and some less frequent conditions (idiopathic retroperitoneal fibrosis, antiphospholipid syndrome, hemolytic-uremic syndrome, etc.) is associated with vascular endothelial damage, increase in certain coagulation and antifibrinolytic factors, decrease in anticoagulation proteins, dyslipidemia, hypoalbuminemia, changes in platelet membranes, hemo- and peritoneal dialysis and heparin treatment, increased microRNAs and circulating microparticles, antiphospholipid antibodies, nephrotic syndrome, anemia with high platelet count, and so on. Nevertheless, the same patients have substantially increased risk of bleeding due to platelet dysfunction and intake of certain medications (antiaggregants, heparin and low-molecular weight heparins, and anemia). The aim of this review is to present the main thrombo-embolic risk factors in a wide variety of patients with renal diseases, including chronic glomerulonephritis (primary and secondary), chronic renal disease, and idiopathic retroperitoneal fibrosis. We have evaluated the risk factors for arterial and venous thromboses in a wide variety of renal patients with both glomerular and non-glomerular diseases, including the presence of nephrotic syndrome, inborn and acquired coagulation defects (i.e., factor V Leiden, MTHFR gene mutation, 20210 prothrombin gene mutation, and antiphospholipid antibodies), corticosteroid treatment, and dyslipidemia. We are describing the results of these investigations and suggesting prophylactic anticoagulant strategies in such patients. Multiple risk factors influence the coagulation system in renal disease leading to both hypercoagulation and hemorrhagic diathesis. Therefore, renal patients should be thoroughly investigated for coagulation abnormalities, especially if pathogenic (i.e., corticosteroid and immunosuppressive) and anticoagulation treatment is to be initiated. Moreover, the doses of anticoagulant/antiaggregant and hemostatic medications should be considered carefully, having in mind the underlying diseases and risk factors, renal function, and concomitant treatment.

Keywords: thromboembolism, glomerulonephritis, retroperitoneal fibrosis, coagulation, anticoagulation

1. Introduction

Patients with renal diseases are prone to both thrombosis and bleeding, as they have profound changes in all three classic components of coagulation, defined approximately 150 years ago by Virchow: blood flow, vessel wall (endothelial injury), and coagulation properties of the blood (e.g., coagulation and fibrinolytic systems, platelets). In this aspect, chronic kidney disease (CKD) is a unique state with the simultaneous presentation of both thrombophilia and hemorrhagic diathesis.

The *prothrombotic state* in CKD, glomerular diseases (including systemic lupus and vasculitis), and some less frequent conditions (idiopathic retroperitoneal fibrosis (RPF), antiphospholipid syndrome (APS), hemolytic-uremic syndrome, etc.) is associated with [1–10]:

- vascular endothelial damage,
- increase in certain coagulation and antifibrinolytic factors,
- decrease in anticoagulation proteins,
- dyslipidemia,
- nephrotic syndrome and hypoalbuminemia,
- changes in platelet membranes,
- hemo- and peritoneal dialysis (PD) and heparin treatment,
- increased microRNAs and circulating microparticles (MPs),
- antiphospholipid antibodies,
- anemia with high platelet count, and so on.

Nevertheless, the same patients have *substantially increased risk of bleeding* due to [6–8]:

- platelet dysfunction,
- impaired platelet-vessel wall interactions,
- intake of certain medications (antiaggregants, heparin and low-molecular weight heparins (LMWHs), and anemia),
- vascular wall abnormalities,
- accompanying disease and conditions (i.e., anemia, myeloma, amyloidosis, etc.), and
- dialysis treatment.

2. Overview of coagulation abnormalities in renal diseases

Renal diseases have high prevalence among the population worldwide. On the other hand, thrombo-embolic complications, including large vascular thromboses (stroke and myocardial infarction and peripheral arterial disease), deep vein thrombosis (DVT) and pulmonary embolism (PE), venous access thromboses, placental thromboses, thromboses of retinal vein and/or arteries, and so on, are also very prevalent in adults, especially in the groups > 65 years of age. Due to the specific metabolic, vascular, plasma, and platelet changes and at the background of inborn hemostasis and bleeding disorders, renal diseases can be associated with both hypercoagulation (thrombophilia) and bleeding (hemorrhagic diathesis) [3–7]. Moreover, CKD itself, irrespective of its underlying cause, is a major risk factor for thromboembolic complications [4–8, 10].

2.1. Hypercoagulation

The underlying mechanism of *thrombophilia* in renal disease, including CKD and chronic renal failure (CRF), is associated with platelet abnormalities, coagulation cascade changes, anemia, endothelial dysfunction and damage, circulating microparticles and miRNAs, atherosclerosis, inborn (protein S and C and anti-thrombin III deficiency, 20210 prothrombin gene mutation, methylene tetrahydrofolate reductase (MTHFR) gene mutation, factor V Leiden, etc.) and acquired thrombophilia (antiphospholipid syndrome and nephrotic syndrome), intake of certain medications and illicit drugs (including corticosteroids, cocaine, heparin, etc.), and dialysis [6–8, 10]. All these changes could be summarized as: increased platelet activation/aggregation, activated coagulation and decreased endogenous anticoagulation, and decreased fibrinolysis.

2.1.1. Platelet abnormalities/dysfunction

In catabolic patients, especially on peritoneal dialysis, it has been shown that decreased plasma levels of nitric oxide (NO) and L-arginine are associated with increased platelet aggregation. Moreover, the increase of phosphatidylserine on platelet surface in CKD/CRF leads to activation of caspase-3 and binding of factor V with subsequent thrombin formation. Besides, CKD/CRF patients have increased PAC-1 fibrinogen receptor and circulating P-selectin that lead to formation of platelet-leukocyte aggregates and formation of free oxygen radicals leading to increased tendency toward thrombosis.

In dialysis, especially in peritoneal dialysis (PD), hypoalbuminemia is thought to lead to platelet activation.

It should be mentioned that in CKD/CRF, there are other functional platelet abnormalities associated with increased bleeding tendency, including decreased GPIb on platelet surface, suppressed function of GPIIb/IIIa, inhibited platelet aggregation changes in platelet alpha-granules, changes in calcium levels, abnormalities in prostaglandin and arachidonic acid metabolism, increased circulating fibrinogen fragments, uremic toxins that inhibit both thrombopoiesis in the bone marrow and platelet aggregation, amyloid deposition in the vessel walls and bone marrow inhibits platelet-vessel wall interactions and thrombopoiesis, and so on.

Paradoxically, in patients with CRF, the described platelet adhesion defects are accompanied by hypercoagulation due to endothelial damage and increased coagulation factor levels and activity plus decreased fibrinolytic activity.

2.1.2. *Coagulation cascade abnormalities*

CKD/CRF is a well-known pro-inflammatory state with increased acute-phase proteins (including C-reactive protein [CRP] and coagulation factors, i.e., fibrinogen) and interleukin 6 (IL-6), increased plasma tissue factor (TF) levels, increased nuclear factor kappa-B (NF-kB) and PAR-1 receptor, decreased levels and activity of anti-thrombin III. On the other hand, in CKD and CRF, marked activation of rennin-angiotensin-aldosterone system (RAAS) is described with increase in plasma fibrinogen levels and plasminogen activator inhibitor 1 (PAI-1). The latter mechanism is associated with both prothrombotic state and progression of CKD itself and closes a vicious circle of CKD—hypertension and prothrombotic state—CKD progression and thrombosis, leading to further worsening of CKD and thromboses.

In (auto)immune renal diseases, hypercoagulability state is due to increased acute-phase proteins and coagulation cascade factors plasma levels and vascular wall/endothelial abnormalities with or without concomitant platelet count and/or activation changes.

2.1.3. *Anemia*

Anemia in CKD is due to erythropoietin deficiency, iron deficiency due to malabsorption of iron + chronic gastrointestinal tract (GIT) bleeding + intake of medications + folic acid and B12 deficiency + chronic inflammation and hypercatabolic state. Anemia is associated with both thrombophilia (especially in cases with chronic bleeding and compensatory increase in platelet count) and bleeding tendency (due to affection of platelet-vessel wall interaction, decreased release of adenosine diphosphate (ADP) and decreased scavenging of NO, inactivation of prostaglandin I2 [PGI2]). The correction of anemia with erythropoiesis-stimulating agents is also a double-edged sword; it can lead to the correction of bleeding tendency but it could also increase blood viscosity and arterial pressure and lead to increased incidence of stroke and myocardial infarction.

2.1.4. *Endothelial dysfunction and damage*

Endothelial dysfunction and damage in CKD/CRF is associated with changes in tissue plasminogen activator (tPA), PAI-1 and von Willebrand factor (vWF) secretion and in NO synthesis and secretion. These alterations, as it has been mentioned above, can lead to both hyper- and hypocoagulation due to impaired platelet-vessel wall interaction and changes in vascular tone and inflammatory response (including oxygen radical generation and scavenging).

Another suspected culprit for the development of hypercoagulation in CKD/CRF is hyperhomocysteinemia leading to endothelial damage, changes in fibrin formation tPA secretion, increase in PAI1, and metalloproteinase-9 activity.

http://dx.doi.org/10.5772/intechopen.68486

In renal transplantation (RT) patients, the calcineurin inhibitor and/or azathioprine-induced endothelial damage + corticosteroid treatment could lead to hypercoagulation and venous thromboembolism (VTE).

In illicit drug users, the intake of heroin, cocaine, and amphetamines has been associated with both renal damage (marked vasoconstriction, rhabdomyolysis, and glomerulosclerosis) and thrombosis (thrombotic microangiopathy due to endothelial damage) [11]. Moreover, in heroin-dependent subjects, drug-induced antiphospholipid antibodies with thrombo-embolic complications have been described [11, 12].

2.1.5. Microparticles

Microparticles (MPs) are cell-membrane residues containing phospholipids (phosphatidylserine) and proteins (tissue factor, residues of cell receptors, etc.). MPs are formed during different processes, such as cell development, differentiation and aging, inflammation, and cell death. MPs are known to have pro-coagulant effects due to phosphatidylserine and TF. Sometimes MPs are associated with small and presumed non-coding single-stranded RNA molecules, called microRNAs (miRNAs). These miRNAs are known to participate in post-transcriptional gene modulation. It has been discovered that they can modulate platelet function via the P2Y12 receptor and/or the VAMP8 or via influencing the platelet mRNA regulation.

2.1.6. Atherosclerosis and vascular injury

Atherosclerosis is a well-known and independent risk factor for the development of large vascular incidents (including stroke and myocardial infarction). All CKD/CRF patients, especially in the presence of nephrotic syndrome, chronic inflammation, and corticosteroid treatment, have accelerated atherosclerosis development. Moreover, the co-morbidities in atherosclerosis and CKD/CRF patients (diabetes, hypertension, obesity, and dyslipidemia) also predispose to both arterial and venous thromboses, probably via following mechanisms: endothelial/vessel wall injury and platelet dysfunction. Microalbuminuria, a marker of endothelial injury, is associated with the risk for the development of both arterial and venous thromboses.

2.1.7. Hypercoagulation in glomerulonephritis

In patients with glomerular diseases, hypercoagulation is associated with four major factors: nephrotic syndrome, vasculitis and vascular wall inflammation, and medications (corticosteroids and cyclosporine A).

The nephrotic syndrome leads to hypercoagulation due to imbalance between pro-and anti-coagulation factors: decreased protein C and S and anti-thrombin III, decreased fibrinolysis, and increased coagulation factor plasma levels. The development of DVT and/or PE is one of the major complications of the nephrotic syndrome. The latter substantially increases the risk for venous thromboembolism.

Vasculitis/vascular wall inflammation in systemic and renal vasculitis, including antineutrophil cytoplasmic antibody (ANCA)-positive cases, leads to hypercoagulation due to structural changes in the vessel wall, endothelial damage, and dysfunction and activation of coagulation cascade. Moreover, high platelet count is observed in acute and chronic inflammation.

Rarely, in patients with systemic vasculitis, parenchymal organ bleeding has been described, associated with microvascular damage and development of small cracks filled with blood (peliosis).

The intake of corticosteroids is associated with increased platelet count and aggregability, increase in coagulation factors plasma levels, and in acute-phase proteins. On the other hand, corticosteroid treatment is associated with the development of GIT hemorrhages due to the inhibition of prostaglandin synthesis. Cyclosporine A treatment can lead to endothelial cell damage with the subsequent development of hypercoagulation and thrombotic microangiopathy. Cocaine, amphetamines, and heroin also affect endothelial cells and can lead to the development of thrombotic microangiopathy.

2.1.8. Antiphospholipid antibodies (APLs)

These autoantibodies are directed against negatively charged plasma or membrane phospholipids and/or phospholipid binding proteins and/or phospholipid-protein complexes. They are the major laboratory criterion for the classification of the antiphospholipid syndrome. APLs affect not only the coagulation system but also endothelial function and platelets. They are known to cause both arterial and venous thromboses, low platelet count, reproductive failure, and accelerated atherosclerosis.

Their determination in renal diseases is crucial because the results can affect both the diagnosis (particularly in chronic glomerulonephritis patients in whom systemic lupus erythematosus (SLE) is suspected) and the treatment, especially at the background of other thrombophilic factors, such as nephrotic syndrome, corticosteroid treatment, vasculitis, dyslipidemia, and diabetes.

The suspected pathogenic mechanism of the pro-coagulant action of APL and the development of vascular injury are [13–18]:

- inhibition of the activated protein C,
- activation of the tissue factor,
- inhibition of anti-thrombin III,
- damage of the membrane annexin V,
- inhibition of the anticoagulant activity of beta-2-glycoprotein-I (b2GPI),
- inhibition of fibrinolysis,
- endothelial cell activation,
- increased expression of adhesion molecules on endothelial cells and leukocyte adhesion to the vascular endothelium,
- neutrophil leukocyte activation and degranulation,
- increased platelet activation and aggregation,

- increased adhesion of b2GPI and prothrombin to the cell membranes,
- effect on endothelial cell apoptosis,
- inhibition of the prostacyclin secretion from endothelial cells, and
- accelerated atherosclerosis.

On the other hand, APLs have several anticoagulant effects, associated with inhibition of factor IX and X activation and of the conversion of prothrombin to thrombin [14]. The factors that modulate the pro- and anticoagulant effects of ALA probably are the phospholipids that bind APL and the antigenic specificity of the latter.

The development of thrombosis in APL-positive patients has been explained by the so-called *second-hit theory*: the presence of APL (first hit) itself is not sufficient for the generation of thrombus but when a second abnormality develops (i.e., endothelial damage, platelet dysfunction, etc.), thrombus may be formed [14]. Moreover, APL could represent the second hit—at the background of inborn or acquired thrombophilia: factor V Leiden or prothrombin gene mutation, MTHFR, protein C/S or anti-thrombin deficiency, nephritic syndrome, chronic renal failure, chronic endothelial damage or dysfunction in chronic inflammation, corticosteroid treatment, and so on. In APS patients, we showed increased platelet activation markers' expression [16]. Some of the APS patients have other underlying inborn coagulation deficiency [18]: protein S/C or anti-thrombin III deficiency, factor V Leiden, 20210 prothrombin gene mutation. This fact supports the described second-hit theory.

2.1.9. *Heparin-induced thrombocytopenia type II (HIT II)*

HIT II is associated with the heparin-induced synthesis of platelet-activating antibodies against the complex heparin-platelet factor 4. It is observed in 0.5–5% of all heparin-treated patients. In such patients, platelet levels are low but thrombo-embolic complications (usually venous thromboses) appear due to platelet activation.

2.2. Bleeding tendency (hemorrhagic diathesis)

The underlying mechanisms of *hemorrhagic diathesis* in renal diseases, CKD and CRF, are associated with platelet dysfunction, uremic toxins, dialysis membranes, impaired platelet-vessel wall interaction, anemia, and intake of certain medications (including aspirin and non-steroid anti-inflammatory drugs [NSAIDs], anticoagulants, antiaggregants, and antibiotics) [6–8].

2.2.1. *Platelet dysfunction*

The main cause of hemorrhagic diathesis in chronic renal diseases, CKD and CRF, are platelet abnormalities, including low platelet count in CKD/CRF due to bone marrow suppression and/or immune thrombocytopenia, changes in alpha-granules with increased adenosine triphosphate (ATP)/ADP ratio, and reduced serotonin content, dysregulation of arachidonate and prostaglandin synthesis and degradation (mainly decreased thromboxane A2), increased plasma levels of fibrinogen fragments.

The changes in alpha-granules are associated with decreased platelet factor 4, fibronectin B, platelet-derived growth factor, vWF, fibrinogen, serotonin, factors V and XIII, transforming growth factor B, and so on.

2.2.2. Uremic toxins

In CKD and CRF, several uremic toxins affect platelet degranulation and adhesion: phenol and phenolic acid, guanidinosuccinic acid, middle molecules (molecular weight of 500–3000 Da). Moreover, uremic toxins inhibit thrombopoiesis in the bone marrow. Low calcium levels in CKD/CRF can also contribute to hypocoagulation. Hemodialysis (HD) and peritoneal dialysis have dual and controversial effect on bleeding and coagulation. Both methods are associated with hypercatabolism, pro-inflammatory state, malabsorption, anemia, and low calcium that could cause both bleeding and hypercoagulation. Moreover, the administration of heparin could cause both bleeding and thromboses (HIT II).

Parathyroid hormone (PTH) has been shown to inhibit platelet aggregation (at least *in vitro*). In hemodialysis, the dialysis membrane can lead to platelet activation and aggregation, but the removal of uremic toxins can (at least partially) correct coagulation abnormalities.

And, finally, circulating fibrinogen fragments that are elevated in CKD/CRF can competitively bind to GPIIb/IIIa platelet receptors and decrease platelet adhesion and aggregation.

2.2.3. Dialysis membranes

Dialysis membranes lead to persistent platelet activation (including increased number and percentage of P-selectin/CD63-positive circulating platelets), formation of platelet-leukocyte (with the generation of free oxygen radicals), and platelet-erythrocyte aggregates [9]. The process of platelet activation is dependent on the type of dialyzer membranes used (more pronounced in cellulose diacetate and polysulfone membranes and less severe in EVAL membranes). The persistent chronic inflammation and hypercatabolism in CRF/CKD also contribute to hypercoagulation. Yet, some patients on dialysis develop thrombocytopenia with bleeding diathesis.

The dialysis (HD and continuous ambulatory peritoneal dialysis [CAPD]) is known to correct, at least partially, the coagulation abnormalities in CKD/CRF.

2.2.4. Platelet-vessel wall interaction

Platelet-vessel wall interactions are associated with the binding of platelets to vWF and fibrinogen on endothelial surface and the activation of platelet receptors (GPIb and GPIIa/IIIb). In the hypercatabolic environment of CKD/CRF, significant decrease of platelet GPIb has been reported, along with decreased platelet binding to fibrinogen and vWF (plus decreased vWF levels), decreased activation of GPIIa/IIIb [6]. The impaired platelet adhesion is thought to be caused by dialyzable uremic toxins, as dialysis corrects the described abnormalities. Moreover, the administration of vWF-containing cryoprecipitates and of desmopressin (known to stimulate endothelial release of vWF) has been shown to ameliorate platelet-vessel wall interactions. And finally, the changes in vascular tone in response to vasoactive substances (nitric oxide and prostacyclin) associated with the accumulation of uremic toxins also contribute to the impairment of platelet-endothelial interactions.

2.2.5. Anemia

Anemia is known to directly influence bleeding because red blood cells lead to platelet aggregation and stimulate ADP release and PGI2 inactivation. Moreover, in patients with CKD/CRF, the infusion of red blood cells and/or the correction of erythrocyte levels with erythropoiesis-stimulating agents and iron lead to reduction of bleeding time. On the other hand, one should not forget that the correction of anemia increases the risk for major vascular incidents (myocardial infarction and stroke).

2.2.6. Drugs and medications

In patients with renal diseases, many drugs may cause severe bleeding episodes, even life-threatening, due to changes in the drug clearance and drug accumulation anticoagulants: direct thrombin inhibitors, aspirin and non-steroid anti-inflammatory drugs [NSAIDs], interaction with platelet membranes (beta-lactam antibiotics, inhibition of cyclooxygenase (aspirin and NSAIDs).

In patients with opioid dependence, Savona et al. [19] describe heroin-induced autoimmune thrombocytopenia. Moreover, in heroin and cocaine/amphetamine dependency, the development of endothelial drug injury may lead to thrombotic microangiopathy with both thromboses and bleeding [11].

The underlying mechanisms for the development of hypercoagulation and bleeding tendency in CKD are summarized in **Table 1**.

The main clinical presentations of thromboses in renal diseases are summarized in **Table 2**.

Hypercoagulation	Bleeding
Platelet activation	Platelet defects
Vascular endothelial damage	Impaired platelet-vessel wall activations
Microparticles and micro RNA	Vascular damage
Oxidative stress	Oxidative stress
Increased von Willebrand factor (vWF)	Defective binding of vWF to GPIIb/IIIa
Increased	Defective prostacyclin and NO synthesis
Increased factor XIIa and VIIa and thrombin formation	Anemia
Decreased protein C and protein S and anti-thrombin III	
Increased tissue factor and acute-phase proteins: fibrinogen, CRP	

Hypercoagulation	Bleeding
Decreased tissue plasminogen activator (tPA)	Increased tPA
Increased plasminogen activator inhibitor 1 (PAI1)	Decreased PAI1
Uremic toxins	Uremic toxins
Increased rennin-angiotensin-aldosterone (RAAS) activity	
Antiphospholipid antibodies	
- Pro-thrombotic gene mutations	Medications
- Factor V Leiden	- Beta-lactam antibiotics
- MTHFR	- Aspirin and NSAIDs
- 20210 prothrombin gene mutation	- Anticoagulants
- Protein C, S, and anti-thrombin deficiency	- Antiaggregants
Nephrotic syndrome	Amyloidosis, myeloma
Anemia	Anemia
Atherosclerosis: dyslipidemia, diabetes, arterial hypertension, peripheral vascular disease	Vasculitis
Corticosteroid treatment, cyclosporine A, cocaine	Corticosteroid treatment
Heparin-induced thrombocytopenia type II	
Hemodialysis and peritoneal dialysis	Hemodialysis and peritoneal dialysis

Table 1. Factors leading to coagulation abnormalities in renal diseases.

Hypercoagulation
- Venous thromboembolism (deep venous thrombosis [DVT] and/or pulmonary embolism [PE]).
- Major vascular incidents (myocardial infarction and/or stroke, peripheral arterial disease).
- Hemodialysis vascular access and/or central venous access thrombosis.
- Peripheral vascular access thrombosis.
- Thrombotic microangiopathy.
Bleeding
- Skin and linings: ecchymoses, epistaxis, gingival bleeding, gastrointestinal bleeding, subungual hematoma, genital bleeding, hematuria, hemoptysis, and skin hemorrhages (petechiae, purpura, and suffusions).
- Intracranial hemorrhage (epidural, subdural, subarachnoid, and intracranial).
- Vascular access bleeding.
- Parenchymal organ bleeding (including peliosis).

Table 2. Clinical presentation of coagulation abnormalities in renal diseases.

http://dx.doi.org/10.5772/intechopen.68486

3. Coagulation abnormalities and their clinical presentation in different renal diseases

3.1. Glomerulonephritis, systemic lupus, and vasculitis

Christiansen et al. [2] examined the risk of VTE in 128,096 Danish patients hospitalized for VTE for the period 1980–2010 (78,623 with DVT and 54,473 with PE) and compared them with 642,426 age- and gender-matched control and found that kidney disease is associated with higher OR for VTE (range between 1.41 for hypertensive nephropathy and 2.89 for nephritic syndrome), with the association being stronger during the first 3 months after the diagnosis of CKD but remaining elevated for the following 5 years. Therefore, the authors concluded that patients with chronic nephropathies are at increased risk for VTE, especially in cases of nephritic syndrome and glomerulonephritis.

In 182 patients with idiopathic glomerulonephritis (125 male and 57 female, mean age 35.6 ± 13.4 years), hospitalized for the period 2000–2005, we observed thrombotic complications in 27: stroke in 6, myocardial infarction in 12, DVT in 15, PE in 7 (the sum is more than 27 because several patients had more than 1 thrombotic complications) [15 and unpublished data]. The main risk factors for the development of thrombotic incidents were nephrotic syndrome (OR 3.220), corticosteroid treatment (OR 2.617), and renal failure (OR 1.51). **Figure 1** shows the typical S1Q3T3 electrocardiography (ECG) changes in a male patient with membranous glomerulonephritis and pulmonary embolism.

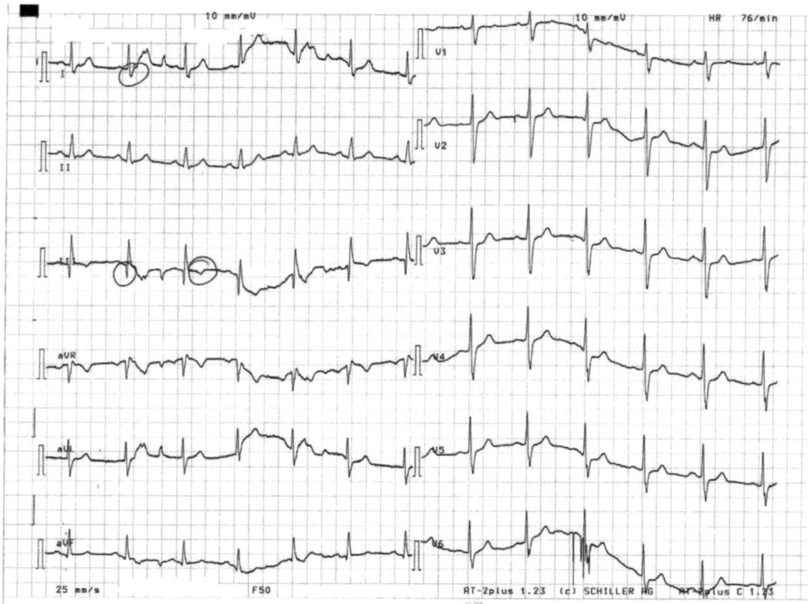

Figure 1. ECG of a patient with idiopathic membranous glomerulonephritis with nephrotic syndrome and pulmonary embolism (PE). Typical S1Q3T3 changes.

In 106 patients with SLE (63 with biopsy-proven lupus nephritis [LN]), 7 male and 56 female, mean age 37.4 ± 10.4 years; 43 without clinical/laboratory data for renal involvement, 7 male and 36 female, mean age 44.1 ± 17.8 years) for the period 2000–2005, we observed thrombotic complications in 34 patients (32.1%) (7/43 without LN and 27/63 with LN) [15]. Following thrombotic incidents were observed:

- Arterial thromboses: coronary incidents in 3, stroke/transient ischemic attack in 8.
- Venous thromboses: DVT in 13, PE in 6, vena axillaris/subclavia thrombosis in 1, vena cava inferior thrombosis in 1.
- Reproductive failure in 8.
- Disseminated intravascular coagulation in 3.
- Thrombotic microangiopathy in 1.

The sum of incidents is more than 34 because several patients had more than 1 thrombotic complication.

The development of thrombotic complications correlated with the presence of positive IgG and IgM anticardiolipin antibody (ACL) and IgG b2GPI (but not IgM b2GPI) and their levels, the presence of APS, the serum cryoglobulin levels and showed weak correlation with the presence of vasculitis (thrombosis+/vasculitis+ 11/106 patients vs. thrombosis−/vasculitis+ 6/106 patients, $r = 0.306$, $p = 0.01$).

For the total population of SLE patients (with and without LN), the development of thrombotic complications correlated with systemic lupus erythematosus disease activity index (SLEDAI) (mean SLEDAI in thrombotic patients 16.2 ± 8.7 vs. 7.6 ± 3.9 for non-thrombotic patients, $r = 0.566$, $p = 0.0001$) and systemic lupus collaborating clinics (SLICC) indices (mean SLICC 2.9 ± 2, vs. 0.7 ± 1.1, respectively, $r = 0.593$, $p = 0.0001$), with the presence of renal involvement (27/63 with LN vs. 7/43 without LN, $\chi^2 = 8.286$, $r = 0.380$, $p = 0.004$).

For the total SLE population (with and without LN), following markers for increased thrombotic risk were identified: arthritis/arthralgiae, serositis, central nervous system involvement, renal involvement, nephritic urinary sediment, nephrotic syndrome, positive IgG and IgM ACL and IgG (but not IgM) b2GPI antibodies, APS, corticosteroid treatment, and vasculitis (**Table 3**).

Marker	OR (95% CI)	*p*
Arthritis/arthralgiae	5.167 (1.433–18.627)	0.007
Serositis	2.537 (1.062–6.059)	0.034
Central nervous system involvement	9 (3.321–24.388)	0.0001
Renal involvement (LN, nephritic urinary sediment, proteinuria, nephrotic syndrome)	3.857 (1.49–9.984)	0.004
Positive IgG ACL	16.8 (6.083–46.398)	0.0001

Marker	OR (95% CI)	*p*
Positive IgM ACL	6.5 (2.305–18.326)	0.0001
Positive IgG b2GPI	5.672 (1.175–28.251)	0.025
APS	148.455 (18.171–1212.827)	<0.0001
Corticosteroid treatment	3.220 (1.576–6.49)	0.0001
Vasculitis	5.261 (1.747–15.838)	0.001

Table 3. Markers of thrombotic risk in 106 patients with SLE [15].

In the investigated LN patients, the development of thrombotic complications correlated with the presence of vasculitis, the duration and the number of SLE criteria, the central nervous system involvement, oral ulcerations, arthritis/arthralgiae, LN histological activity index, the amount of proteinuria, serum cryoglobulin levels, the levels and positivity of IgG and IgM ACL, the mean IgG b2GPI levels, SLEDAI and SLICC, APS, and inversely correlated with serum IgG levels (lower in more severe nephrotic syndrome).

In LN patients, the following markers of increased thrombotic risk were identified: oral ulcerations and vasculitis, positive ANCA, central nervous system involvement, nephrotic syndrome, positive IgG and IgM ACL and IgG b2GPI, hypocomplementemia C3, APS, and corticosteroid treatment (**Table 4**).

The results of our studies in APS patients with and without SLE [16] showed correlation between CD63 expression and activated partial thromboplastin time (aPTT), CD61 expression and IgG and IgM ACL, and b2GPI, CD42a, and b2GPI.

Marker	OR (95% CI)	*p*
Oral ulcerations	2.0 (1.97–3.79)	0.001
Central nervous system involvement	10.54 (3.094–35.905)	0.0001
Nephrotic syndrome	2.448 (0.869–6.895)	0.05
ANCA	3.008 (1.068–8.473)	0.035
Positive IgG ACL	18.229 (5.097–65.127)	<0.0001
Positive IgM ACL	7.563 (1.848–30.955)	0.002
Positive IgG b2GPI	5.238 (1.057–25.966)	0.036
Hypocomplementemia C3	2.020 (1.204–3.387)	0.015
APS	5.5 (2.939–10.294)	<0.0001
Corticosteroid treatment	3.077 (1.507–6.283)	0.01
Vasculitis	17.5 (2.053–149.153)	0.001

Table 4. Markers of increased thrombotic risk in 63 LN patients [15].

The results of our investigations on the platelet activation markers in female patients with complicated pregnancy [18], including edema-proteinuria-hypertension (EPH) gestosis, revealed that these patients have increased anticardiolipin and beta-2-glycoprotein I antibodies, and the levels of ACL correlate with CD63 expression (marker of platelet degranulation). Some of the APL-positive patients also had inborn coagulation defects (i.e., factor V Leiden 20210 prothrombin gene mutation and MTHFR gene mutation).

3.2. Retroperitoneal fibrosis

Idiopathic retroperitoneal fibrosis (RPF) is a rare autoimmune fibrosing disease associated with the development of fibrous tissue and/or chronic inflammatory infiltrates (**Figure 2**) in the retroperitoneal space that envelops the aorta, iliac vessels, and ureters (**Figure 3**) [20]. In approximately 15% of the patients, extra-abdominal fibrosis is observed. In some RPF patients with vascular involvement, thrombotic incidents have been described [20]. For the period 1998–2017, we followed 33 patients with idiopathic retroperitoneal fibrosis (25 male and 8 female). Overall 17 patients had thrombotic incidents: iliac/femoral vein thrombosis in 8, vena cava inferior thrombosis in 4, portal vein thrombosis in 2, infiltration (with or without thrombosis) of the inferior mesenteric artery and its branches (**Figure 4**) in 3, aortic aneurism with thrombosis (**Figure 5**) in 2, DVT with or without PE in 5 (the sum of events is more

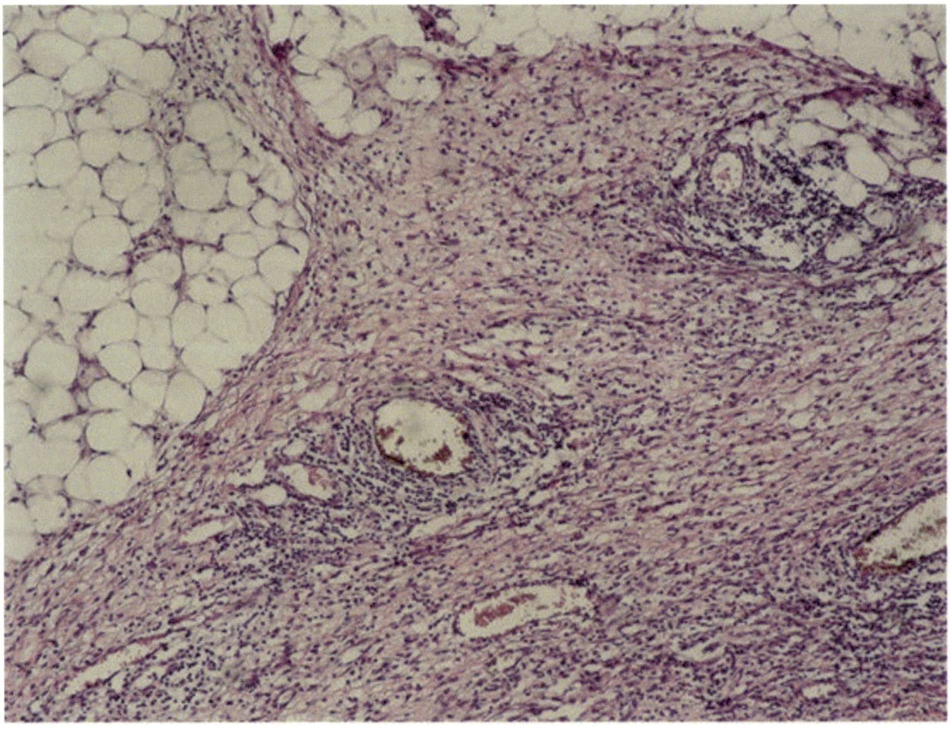

Figure 2. Biopsy specimen of retroperitoneal infiltrates in a patient with idiopathic retroperitoneal fibrosis (RPF)—inflammatory infiltrate with abundance of lymphocytes and fibrous tissue.

http://dx.doi.org/10.5772/intechopen.68486

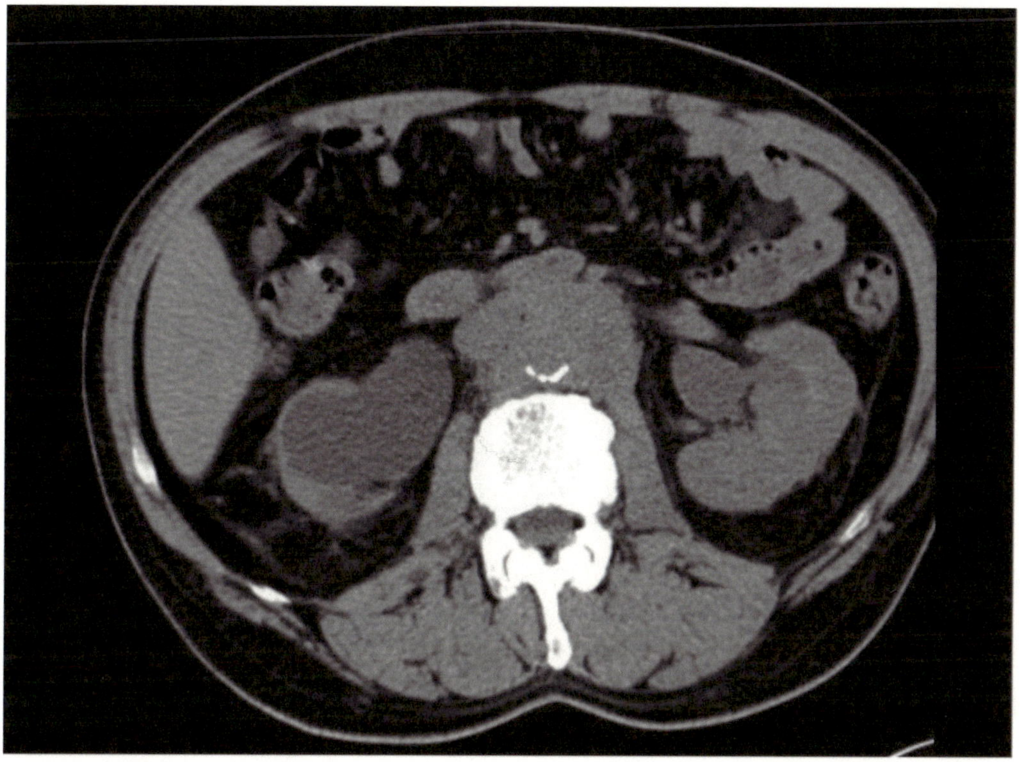

Figure 3. CT image of a patient with idiopathic RPF. Bilateral hydronephrosis and retroperitoneal infiltrates that envelop the aorta, iliac vessels, and ureters.

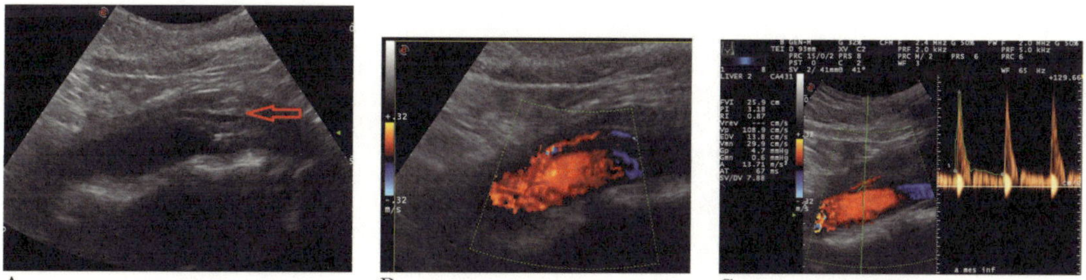

A B C

Figure 4. Abdominal ultrasound in a patient with idiopathic RPF (arrow) with involvement of the abdominal aorta and inferior mesenteric artery (A and B), no Doppler data for stenosis of the inferior mesenteric artery (C). *Courtesy of Dr. R. Krasteva-Lolova.*

than 17 because several patients had more than 1 thrombotic complication). In one patient, the DVT episodes with varico- and hyrdocele (**Figure 6**) were the first manifestation of RPF. The underlying mechanism of thrombosis in RPF is associated with vascular wall changes, endothelial dysfunction in chronic inflammation, corticosteroid/azathioprine treatment, and immune phenomena (including APL).

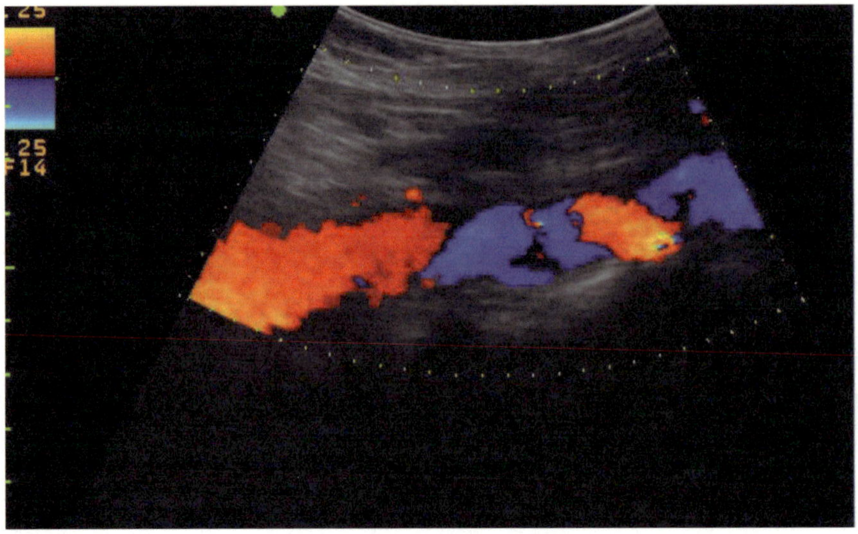

Figure 5. Abdominal Doppler ultrasound of a patient with idiopathic RPF with aortic aneurism.

3.3. Drug abuse

The intake of illicit drugs (including heroin, cocaine, and amphetamines) has been reported to be associated with thrombotic incidents. The possible underlying mechanisms of thrombosis are overdose with rhabdomyolysis with or without acute renal failure and vascular damage; drug-induced endothelial cell injury with thrombotic microangiopathy; platelet and coagulation

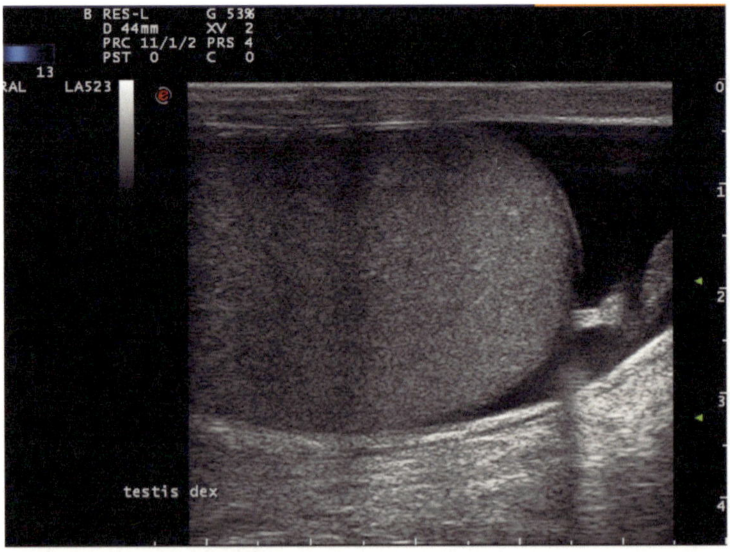

Figure 6. Ultrasound examination of the testicles (right testicle) of a male patient with idiopathic RPF manifesting with femoro-popliteal thrombosis and hydrocele.

abnormalities due to chronic inflammation, drug- and infection-induced APL [11, 12, 15, 19]. In a group of 15 heroin abusers (12 male and 3 female, mean age 23.9 ± 4.2 years), we observed renal involvement in 6 [15]. One of the patients with biopsy-proven renal involvement (chronic tubulo-interstitial nephritis) and negative hepatitis B virus (HBV), hepatitis C virus (HCV), and human immunodeficiency virus (HIV) developed ilio-femoral vein thrombosis and acute renal failure at the background of positive IgG ACL. After the cessation of heroin abuse, ACL levels subsided back to the normal values that suggests heroin-induced autoantibodies. The results of our investigations suggest that in patients with illicit drug abuse, the clinician should be aware of the possible renal and thrombotic complications.

3.4. Chronic kidney disease and chronic renal failure

Chronic renal disease and chronic renal failure are associated with significantly elevated risk for the development of venous thromboembolism due to platelet and coagulation abnormalities, impaired fibrinolysis, and endothelial damage and dysfunction. CKD is classified in five stages according to the degree of glomerular filtration rate (GFR) decrease (**Table 5**). The prevalence of CKD/CRF in adults >20 years of age in the NHANES III study [21] is approximately 11%. This fact shows the social significance of CKD. Having in mind the increased thrombotic risk in mild to moderate CKD patients (1.3–2-fold increase compared to the general population) and end-stage renal disease (2.3-fold compared to the general population), the clinician should be aware of VTE as a possible complication of CKD/CRF and of the need of proper anticoagulation strategy [3, 10].

3.5. Hemodialysis and peritoneal dialysis

As it was mentioned above, dialysis treatment is associated with both thrombosis and increased risk for bleeding episodes [1, 4–7]. The coagulation abnormalities (including the changes in the coagulation pathway, anticoagulation, and fibrinolysis/antifibrinolysis) in hemodialysis (HD) and continuous ambulatory peritoneal dialysis (CAPD) are summarized in **Table 6**. These changes are accompanied by platelet abnormalities and altered platelet-vascular wall interactions [7]. The

Stage	GFR (ml/min/1.72 m² body surface)	Prevalence (USA, NHANES III, adults >20 years of age) (%) [21]
0	>90, Normal GFR, no risk for CKD/CRF, no underlying renal disease or damage	89
1	>90, Persistent microalbuminuria and/or risk for CKD/CRF—underlying renal disease or damage	3.3
2	60–89	3.0
3	30–59	4.3
4	15–29	0.2
5	<15 (or dialysis treatment)	0.2

Table 5. Definition of chronic kidney disease and prevalence in the USA according to the NHANES III [21].

Marker	Hemodialysis	Peritoneal dialysis (CAPD)
Coagulation pathway		
Fibrinogen, factor VII, vWF, tissue factor	↑	↑
Factor II, VIII, IX, X, XII	↓	↑
Prothrombin fragments 1 + 2	↑	↑
Anticoagulation		
Thrombomodulin, tissue factor pathway inhibitor	↑	↑
Protein S	↓	↑
Protein C, anti-thrombin III	↓	-
Fibrinolysis		
Tissue plasminogen activator	↑	↓
Plasminogen activator inhibitor 1	↓	↑
Thrombin activable fibrinolysis inhibitor	-	↑

Table 6. Coagulation abnormalities in hemodialysis and in peritoneal dialysis.

in vitro and *in vivo* studies reveal somewhat contradictive results—patients on dialysis can have both increased and decreased platelet aggregation and the initiation of dialysis partially corrects the pre-existing abnormalities in platelet function, characteristic for CKD/CRF [7, 9]. The degree of anemia and hypoalbuminemia seem to correlate with prolonged bleeding time, and the chronic inflammation seems to increase the thrombotic risk [7]. Heparin treatment in HD can induce both bleeding and thromboses (HIT II). The alterations in NO synthesis also lead to decreased platelet aggregation [7].

A major problem in these patients represents the vascular access thrombosis, especially in diabetics and in patients with systemic connective tissue disease (with or without the APS). Anticoagulation strategies in dialysis treatment are discussed further in the text.

3.6. Renal transplantation

VTE is a frequent complication of renal transplantation (RT). According to the literature, 6–7% of RT patients develop VTE [5, 22], including DVT, PE, graft thrombosis, renal vein thrombosis, and thrombotic microangiopathy [8]. The underlying mechanisms, as discussed earlier, include impaired platelet function and platelet-vessel wall interactions, hypercoagulation at the background of chronic inflammation, corticosteroid treatment and CKD, the effect of calcineurin inhibitors and azathioprine on endothelial function, OKT3, and so on [8].

Luna et al. [5] retrospectively analyzed 577 cadaveric RTs performed for the period 1992–2009, excluding the cases with known hypercoagulability before RT. The incidence of VTE was 6%. The authors evaluated the type of thrombosis according to recipient variables, differences in dialysis within 24 h before transplantation (0 no dialysis, 13.8% dialysis out of hospital, and

4.2% dialysis in hospital; $p = 0.029$) and iliac vascular pathology (10% yes vs. 5% no; $p < 0.04$). The authors suggest that donor-related factors are age >60 years (11% vs. 5%; $p = 0.01$), stroke versus trauma as a cause of death (9.3% vs. 4.7%; $p = 0.049$), and graft atheroma (16.7% yes vs. 5.1% no; $p = 0.042$). The authors also investigated the treatment-associated risk factors tacrolimus versus cyclosporine (7.4% vs. 2.3%; $p = 0.001$) and sequential therapy (10.7% yes vs. 3.3% no; $p = 0.001$), basiliximab (adjusted for donor and recipient age, and graft atheroma). The multivariate analysis revealed that the predictive factors for VTE after RT (increasing the risk for VTE (16-fold)) are stroke donor death (OR 3.88), recipient iliac vascular pathology (OR 2.81), and graft atheroma (OR 3.63).

Poli et al. [22] studied 484 RT and found 7% prevalence of first episode of VTE. The authors investigated the importance of the cessation of oral anticoagulation and found that compared to VTE patients without renal disease the recurrence of VTE in RT patients is very high (50% or 14/28 compared to <10% or 8/84). In RT patients, the authors also find higher levels of homocysteine, circulating fibrinogen fragments 1 + 2 and D-dimer that are characteristic for CKD/CRF patients in general. The authors recommend prolonged oral anticoagulation in RT patients to prevent the risk of VTE recurrence, despite the elevated bleeding risk.

4. Anticoagulation strategies

Due to the high risk of VTE all patients with chronic renal diseases, including glomerulonephritis, systemic connective tissue diseases, and vasculitis with renal involvement, retroperitoneal fibrosis, hemodialysis, should be considered possible candidates for anticoagulation, especially in the presence of coagulation abnormalities (anticoagulation factor deficiency, vasculitis, nephrotic syndrome, and CKD/CRF) and/or predisposing factors (atrial fibrillation, various veins, cardiac and renal failure, etc.). Nevertheless, patients with renal diseases represent significant therapeutic challenge if anticoagulation is needed, because they are prone to both thromboses and hemorrhages and because the gastrointestinal absorption and the renal clearance of certain anticoagulants are altered in CKD/CRF [3].

4.1. Unfractioned heparin and low-molecular weight heparins (LMWHs)

Unfractionated heparin (UFH) is a 3–30 kDA sulphated polysaccharide that binds positively charged surfaces. Its anticoagulant response is mediated by binding to factor IIa and factor Xa. UFH anticoagulant effect is monitored using activated partial thromboplastin time (aPTT). UFH has reticulo-endothelial and, to a lesser extent, renal clearance. Therefore, its clearance in CKD/CRF is unpredictable. UFH doses should be reduced in moderate to severe CRF (creatinine clearance below 30 ml/min) with close monitoring of aPTT (1.5–2x prolongation) in order to prevent over-anticoagulation and severe bleeding episodes [6]. In VTE episodes at the background of CRF, Hughes et al. [3] recommend loading dose of 60 U/kg/h with maintenance dose of 12 U/kg/h. Significant side effects of UFH include bleeding, heparin-induced thrombocytopenia, osteopenia, and alopecia, especially in prolonged administration.

LWMHs are synthetic UFH derivatives with shorter heparin chains and stronger affinity to factor Xa with lower affinity to factor IIa. Their pharmacokinetic profile is more predictable than that of UFH. Moreover, self-administration of the medication is possible. LMWHs have lower affinity and binding to endothelial cells and platelets and no routine monitoring of coagulation parameters is required. The only suitable monitoring parameter is anti-Xa levels that is not routinely used in clinical practice. The most frequent side effects in prolonged administration are HIT, osteopenia, and alopecia, and their incidence is much lower compared to that on UFH.

The LMWHs dose should also be reduced in CRF [3]:

- In glomerular filtration rate (GFR) >40 ml/min, full dose once daily.
- In GFR 30–39 ml/min, 80–90% of the recommended dose once daily.
- In GFR <30 ml/min, 60% of the recommended daily dose twice a day.

To avoid sub- or supradosing, monitoring of anti-Xa levels is advisable in CRF patients with GFR <50 ml/min.

4.2. Warfarin and indirect anticoagulants

Indirect anticoagulants are vitamin K antagonists that inhibit the synthesis of vitamin K-dependent coagulation factors. The routine laboratory marker for the monitoring of their effect is prothrombin time (PT)/international normalized ration (INR). In CRF patients with GFR 30–59 ml/min, the maintenance dose required for stabile PT prolongation is 10% lower than that in non-CRF population and in GFR <30 ml/min, the dose is 20% lower [3]. Moreover, CKD/CRF patients tend to have labile PT/INR and the anticoagulant effect is quite unpredictable. In a review on mechanisms of vascular calcifications, El-Abbadi et al. [23] emphasize that indirect anticoagulants can increase vascular calcifications due to vitamin K inhibition-dependent increase of serum phosphate levels. Another major complication is the warfarin-related nephropathy—unexplained increase in serum creatinine with ≥0.3 mg% after the initiation of warfarin treatment probably due to intraglomerular bleeding and tubular obstruction by erythrocyte casts. This complication is associated with marked increase in mortality in CRF patients.

4.3. Newer oral anticoagulants

These medications are synthetic anti-Xa agents (apixaban and rivaroxaban) or anti-IIa agents (dabigatran and direct thrombin inhibitors). Rivaroxaban and apixaban have approximately 30% renal clearance and their effect in CRF patients is more predictable, whereas dabigatran has mainly renal clearance (85%) and in CRF patients tends to accumulate, and its effect in this population is unpredictable. Therefore, rivaroxaban and apixaban are approved for CRF patients with CFR<30 ml/min (with dose reduction of approximately 50%, the dose of rivaroxaban in CFR 15–49 ml/min is 15 mg/day, and <15 ml/min is contraindicated; the dose of apixaban in GFR 15–29 ml/min is 2.5 mg twice a day) and dabigatran is not approved in patient with GFR<30 ml/min [3]. It should be noted that both rivaroxaban and apixaban (anti-Xa agents) have high protein binding and are metabolized via CYP3A4. Therefore, they should be used with caution in patients with nephrotic syndrome or hypoproteinemia/hypoalbuminemia of other origin and in combination with CYP3A4 inhibitors or inductors.

4.4. Antiaggregants

Aspirin, NSAIDs, and clopidogrel should be used with caution in patients with renal diseases because their anti-platelet effects are unpredictable in GFR <30 ml/min, because CRF patients have significant platelet function abnormalities and frequently are thrombocytopenic and anemic and because their clearance is significantly altered in severe renal impairment. Moreover, NSAIDs and aspirin tend to cause severe, even life-threatening gastrointestinal bleeding episodes, especially at the background of uremic gastro-enteropathy, low platelet count, or corticosteroid treatment.

5. Conclusion

Patients with renal diseases are prone to both thrombosis and bleeding. The prothrombotic state in chronic nephropathies is associated with [6–8] vascular endothelial damage, changes in certain coagulation and antifibrinolytic factors, decrease in anticoagulation proteins, dyslipidemia, hypoalbuminemia, changes in platelet membranes, hemo- and peritoneal dialysis and heparin treatment, increased microRNAs and circulating microparticles, antiphospholipid antibodies, nephrotic syndrome, anemia with high platelet count, and so on. Nevertheless, the same patients have substantially increased risk of bleeding due to platelet dysfunction, and intake of certain medications (antiaggregants, heparin and low-molecular weight heparins, and anemia) [6–8].

In this review, we have presented the main thrombo-embolic risk factors in a wide variety of patients with renal diseases, including chronic glomerulonephritis (primary and secondary), CKD/CRF, idiopathic retroperitoneal fibrosis, and dialysis treatment. We have presented our data on thrombotic incidents in patients with glomerular and non-glomerular diseases and the role of certain prothrombotic factors, such as nephrotic syndrome, inborn and acquired coagulation defects (i.e., factor V Leiden, MTHFR gene mutation, 20210 prothrombin gene mutation, and antiphospholipid antibodies), corticosteroid treatment, and so on. Therapeutic and prophylactic anticoagulation in these patients is influenced by many factors, including the underlying renal disease, renal, hepatic, and cardiac function, co-morbidities and accompanying treatment. Moreover, the doses of anticoagulant/antiaggregant and hemostatic medications should be considered carefully. The best and the safest anticoagulant medications in patients with chronic renal diseases (including glomerulonephritis, vasculitis, and CKD/CRF) at this point seem to be LMWHs followed by UFH in dose regimens in accordance with renal function because of their favorable safety profile, flexible dosing regimen, self-administration, short and predictable action, and the possibility to correct the dose according to GFR.

Abbreviations

ACL	Anticardiolipin antibody
ADP	Adenosine diphosphate
ANCA	Antineutrophil cytoplasmic antibody
APL	Antiphospholipid antibody
APS	Antiphospholipid syndrome
aPTT	Activated partial thromboplastin time
ATP	Adenosine triphosphate
b2GPI	Beta-2-glycoprotein I antibody
CAPD	Continuous ambulatory peritoneal dialysis
CKD	Chronic kidney disease
CRF	Chronic renal failure
CRP	C-reactive protein
CT	Computed tomography
DVT	Deep vein thrombosis
ECG	Electrocardiography
EPH	Edema-proteinuria-hypertension
GFR	Glomerular filtration rate
GIT	Gastrointestinal tract
GP	Glycoprotein
HBV	Hepatitis B virus
HCV	Hepatitis C virus
HD	Hemodialysis
HIT II	Heparin-induced thrombocytopenia type II
HIV	Human immunodeficiency virus
IL-6	Interleukin 6
INR	International normalized ration
LMWH	Low-molecular weight heparin

LN	Lupus nephritis
MPs	Microparticles
MTHFR	Methylene tetrahydrofolate reductase
NF-kB	Nuclear factor kappa-B
NO	Nitric oxide
NSAIDs	Non-steroid anti-inflammatory drugs
PAI-1	Plasminogen activator inhibitor 1
PD	Peritoneal dialysis
PE	Pulmonary embolism
PGI2	Prostaglandin I2
PT	Prothrombin time
PTH	Parathyroid hormone
RAAS	Rennin-angiotensin-aldosterone system
RPF	Retroperitoneal fibrosis
RT	Renal transplantation
SLE	Systemic lupus erythematosus
SLEDAI	Systemic lupus erythematosus disease activity index
SLICC	systemic lupus collaborating clinics
TF	Tissue factor
tPA	Tissue plasminogen activator
UFH	Unfractionated heparin
VTE	Venous thromboembolism
vWF	Von Willebrand factor

Author details

Milena Nikolova-Vlahova*, Marta Petrova Baleva and Petar Krasimirov Nikolov

*Address all correspondence to: milena_i_dani@abv.bg

Medical University, Sofia, Bulgaria

References

[1] Casserly LF, Dember LM. Thrombosis in end-stage renal disease. Seminars in Dialysis. 2003;**16**:245–256. DOI: 10.1046/j.1525-139X.2003.16048.x

[2] Christiansen CF, Schmidt M, Lamberg AL, et al. Kidney disease and risk of venous thromboembolism: A nationwide population-based control study. Journal of Thrombosis and Haemostasis. 2014;**12**:1449–1454. DOI: 10.1111/jth.126

[3] Hughes S, Szeki I, Nash MJ, Thachil J. Anticoagulation in chronic kidney disease patients – the practical aspects. Clinical Kidney Journal. 2014;**7**:442–449. DOI: 10.1093/ckj/sfu080

[4] Jalal DI, Chonchon M, Targher G. Disorders of hemostasis associated with chronic kidney disease. Seminars in Thrombosis and Hemostasis. 2010;**36**:35–40. DOI: 10.1055/s-0030-1248722

[5] Luna E, Cerezo I, Collado G, et al. Vascular thrombosis after kidney transplantation: Predisposing factors and risk index. Transplantation Proceedings. 2010;**42**:2928–2930. DOI: 10.1016/j.transproceed.2010.07.085

[6] Lutz J, Menke J, Sollinger D, et al. Hemostasis in chronic kidney disease. Nephrology Dialysis Transplantation. 2014;**29**:29–40. DOI: 10.1093/ndt/gft209

[7] Malyszko J, Malyszko JS, Mysliewiec M, Buczko W. Hemostasis in chronic renal failure. Roczniki Akademii Medycznej w Bialymstoku. 2005;**50**:126–131

[8] Rabelink TJ, Zwazinga JJ, Koomans HA, Sixma JJ. Thrombosis and hemostasis in renal disease. Kidney International. 1994;**46**; 287–296. DOI: http://dx.doi.org/10.1038/ki.1994.274

[9] Sirolli V, Ballone E, Di Stante S, et al. Cell activation and cellular-cellular interactions during hemodialysis: Effect of dialyzer membrane. International Journal of Artificial Organs. 2002; **25**:529–537. PMID: 121172

[10] Wattanakit K, Cushman M. Chronic kidney disease and venous thromboembolism: epidemiology and mechanisms. Current Opinion in Pulmonary Medicine. 2009**;15:**408–412. DOI: 10.1097/MCP.0b013e32832ee371

[11] Nikolova M, Iliev A. Systemic manifestations and renal involvement in narcotic abuse. Medicinski Pregled. 2002;**15**:5–12

[12] Nikolova M, Liubomirova M, Iliev A, et al. Clinical significance of antinuclear antibodies, anti-neutrophil cytoplasmic antibodies and anticardiolipin antibodies in heroin abusers. Israel Medical Association Journal. 2002;**4**(11 Suppl):908-910. PMID: 12455177

[13] Boyanovsky B. Antiphospholipid syndrome – pathogenic effect and diagnostic significance of antiphospholipid antibodies, protein C and factor V Leiden [thesis]. Sofia: Faculty of Medicine, Medical University; 2000

[14] Levine JS, Branch DW, Rauch J. The antiphospholipid syndrome. New England Journal of Medicine. 2002;**346**:752–763. DOI: 10.1056/NEJMra002974

[15] Nikolova M. Diagnostic and prognostic value of some parameters of immune response in patients with different form of glomerulonephritis [thesis]. Sofia: Faculty of Medicine, Medical University; 2007

[16] Popova D, Nikolov Kr, Baleva M, et al. Platelet activation markers in patients with antiphospholipid syndrome. Revmatologia. 2003;**11**:37–41

[17] Vikentieva E, Baleva M. Antiphospholipid syndrome. Medicinski Pregled. 2006;**42**:5–15

[18] Vikentieva E, Popova D, Savov Al, Nikolova M, et al. Platelet activation markers in patients with complicated pregnancy. Medicinski Pregled. 2005;**41**:74–78

[19] Savona S, Nardi MA, Lennette ET, Karpatkin S. Thrombocytopenic purpura in narcotics addicts. Annals of Internal Medicine. 1985;**102**:737–741. PMID: 2986504

[20] Tzou M, Gazeley DJ, Mason PJ. Retroperitoneal fibrosis. Vascular Medicine. 2014;**19**:407–414. DOI: 10.1177/1358863X14546160

[21] Coresh J, Astor BC, Greene T, et al. Prevalence of chronic kidney disease and decreased kidney function in the adult US population: Third National Health and Nutrition Examination Survey. American Journal of Kidney Diseases. 2003;**41**:1–12. DOI: 10.1053/ajkd.2003.50007

[22] Poli D, Zanazzi M, Antonucci E, et al. High rate of recurrence in renal transplant recipients after a first episode of venous thromboembolism. Transplantation. 2005;**80**:789–793. PMID: 16210966

[23] El-Abbadi M, Giachelli CM. Mechanisms of vascular calcification. Advances in Chronic Kidney Disease. 2007;**14**: 54–66. DOI: 10.1053/j.ackd.2006.10.007

Chapter 6

Venous Thromboembolism in Liver Cirrhosis: An Emerging Issue

Xingshun Qi and Andrea Mancuso

Additional information is available at the end of the chapter

http://dx.doi.org/10.5772/67707

Abstract

Venous thromboembolism (VTE) carries a high morbidity and mortality and leads to a substantial economic burden. From the traditional perspectives, liver cirrhosis tends to bleeding but not VTE. However, modern concepts suggest that liver cirrhosis is also at a risk of VTE. The pooled incidence and prevalence of VTE in liver cirrhosis are 1% (95% confidence interval: 0.7–1.3%) and 1% (95% confidence interval: 0.7–1.2%), respectively. Evidence indicates that a higher international normalized ratio and a lower albumin should be associated with a higher probability of VTE in liver cirrhosis. Additionally, the presence of VTE significantly worsens the outcomes of liver cirrhosis.

Keywords: venous thromboembolism, liver cirrhosis, risk factor, prognosis, epidemiology

1. Introduction: venous thromboembolism

Venous thromboembolism (VTE) consists of deep vein thrombosis (DVT) and pulmonary embolism (PE). VTE is a major public health condition.

First, VTE represents a substantial economic burden in this world. A systematic review of 10 cost-of-illness studies explored the costs in the different regions [1]. The initial VTE costs 3000–9500$ in the United States. The additional inpatient costs are significantly increased with the duration of VTE. In the United States, the VTE over 3, 6, and 12 months costs 5000$, 10,000$, and 33,000$, respectively; by comparison, in the EU, the VTE over 3 and 12 months costs 1800$ and $32,000$, respectively. The additional costs of VTE-related complications are also expensive. The post-thrombotic syndrome costs 426–11,700$, and the heparin-induced thrombocytopenia costs 3118–41,133$.

Second, VTE carries a relatively high incidence. In the United States, the annual incidence of VTE is 1/1000 and is gradually increased with the age [2]. A 25-year population-based study, which was conducted in Olmsted County, Minnesota, United States, found that the annual incidence of VTE was 1.17/1000 and that the annual incidences of DVT and PE were 0.48/1000 and 0.69/1000, respectively [3]. A community-based study, in which 342,000 inhabitants were enrolled between April 1, 1998, and March 31, 1999, in Western France, demonstrated that the annual incidence of VTE was 1.83/1000 (95% confidence interval: 1.69–1.98) and that the annual incidences of DVT and PE were 1.24/1000 (95% confidence interval: 1.12–1.36) and 0.60/1000 (95% confidence interval: 0.52–0.69), respectively [4]. Recently, a new community-based study, in which 367,911 inhabitants were enrolled between March 1, 2013, and February 28, 2014, in Western France, demonstrated that the annual incidence of VTE was significantly decreased to 1.57/1000 (95% confidence interval: 1.44–1.69) [5]. A prospective community-based study, in which 151,923 permanent residents of northeastern metropolitan Perth in Western Australia were followed from October 1, 2003, to October 31, 2004, found that the annual incidence of VTE was 0.83/1000 (95% confidence interval: 0.69–0.97) and that the annual incidences of DVT and PE were 0.52 (95% confidence interval: 0.41–0.63) and 0.31 (95% confidence interval: 0.22–0.40), respectively [6]. Indeed, necropsy examinations demonstrated a higher incidence of VTE. Based on a review of necropsy reports from a Swedish Malmo general hospital, 34.7% (347/994) of necropsy cases had VTE, and 9.4% (93/994) of them had fatal PE [7].

Third, VTE produces a high mortality and is a major cause of death in the general population. A population-based cohort study of 2218 patients with DVT or PE from Olmsted County, Minnesota, demonstrated that the 7-day, 30-day, and 1-year survival rates were 96.2, 94.5, and 85.4% in patients with DVT alone and 59.1, 55.6, and 47.7% in patients with PE with or without DVT [8]. A retrospective review of necropsy data from inpatients at King's College Hospital between January 1991 and December 2000 demonstrated that 5.2% (265/6833) of death cases were attributed to fatal PE [9]. The VTE Impact Assessment Group in Europe (VITAE) estimated that the total number of symptomatic VTE events per annum within the six EU countries, including France, Germany, Italy, Spain, Sweden, and the United Kingdom, were 465,715 (404,664–538,189) DVT cases, 295,982 (242,450–360,363) PE cases, and 370,012 (300,193–483,108) VTE-related deaths [10].

2. Risk factors for the development of VTE

Virchow's triad, which includes vessel injury, blood flow stasis, and hypercoagulopathy, is a classical explanation for the development of VTE [11]. According to the 7th American College of Chest Physicians Conference on Antithrombotic and Thrombolytic Therapy, the major risk factors for VTE included surgery, trauma (major or lower extremity), immobility, paresis, malignancy, cancer therapy (hormonal, chemotherapy, or radiotherapy), previous

VTE, increasing age, pregnancy and the postpartum period, estrogen-containing oral contraception or hormone replacement therapy, selective estrogen receptor modulators, acute medical illness, heart or respiratory failure, inflammatory bowel disease, nephrotic syndrome, myeloproliferative disorders, paroxysmal nocturnal hemoglobinuria, obesity, smoking, varicose veins, central venous catheterization, and inherited or acquired thrombophilia [12]. Currently, accumulated evidence has identified more and more risk factors for the development of VTE. A meta-analysis of 14 studies demonstrated a dose-response relationship between duration of travel and development of VTE [13]. Hippisley-Cox et al. developed and validated the QThrombosis web calculator (www.qthrombosis.org) for predicting the risk of VTE between 1 and 5 years [14]. In the calculator, the information should be provided regarding age, sex, ethnicity, smoking status, varicose vein surgery, chronic kidney disease (stage 4 or 5), cancer, heart failure, chronic obstructive airways disease, Crohn's or ulcerative colitis, previous admission in last 6 months, antipsychotics, and body mass index. For women, some additional information regarding hormone replacement therapy, an oral contraceptive, and tamoxifen is needed. Rogers et al. also conducted a case-crossover study to evaluate the triggers of hospitalization for VTE [15]. A total of 399 subjects with VTE hospitalizations were enrolled from the Health and Retirement Study in the United States. The investigators found that infection was the most frequent trigger of VTE (52.4%) and the use of erythropoiesis stimulating agents was the most strong trigger of VTE (adjusted incidence rate ratio = 9.33, 95% confidence interval: 1.19–73.42). More recently, Tsai et al. [16] also assessed the hospital-level determinants of VTE diagnosis. An interesting finding was that patients treated in urban hospitals had a higher risk of VTE diagnosis than those treated in rural hospitals. Except for the above-mentioned findings in the general population, lots of studies focused on the prediction of VTE in patients with cancer, patients undergoing surgery, and other specific population, which were beyond the scope of the present work.

3. Liver cirrhosis

According to the Global Burden of Disease Study 2010, liver cirrhosis is the 11th leading cause of death and accounts for 50,000 deaths in the United States, 2010 [17]. It is also the 8th leading cause of years of life lost from premature death. According to the Global Burden of Disease Study 2013, liver cirrhosis is the 13th leading cause of global years of life lost [18]. The major complications of liver cirrhosis should be esophageal variceal bleeding and ascites [19–21]. Liver cirrhosis is divided into four major stages according to the two complications. They include stage 1 (neither varices nor ascites), stage 2 (varices without ascites), stage 3 (ascites), and stage 4 (variceal bleeding) [22]. Considering the potential risk of lethal variceal bleeding, a patient with liver cirrhosis is considered to have a bleeding diathesis and is often contraindicated for antithrombotic drugs [23]. At present, emerging evidence suggests that a cirrhotic patient is also at a risk of thrombosis due to the loss of anticoagulant proteins [23]. A nationwide Danish case-control study of 99,444 patients with VTE and 496,872 population controls found a significantly higher risk of VTE in patients with liver cirrhosis (all VTE: risk ratio = 1.74, 95% confidence interval: 1.54–1.95; DVT: risk ratio = 2.02, 95% confidence interval: 1.78–2.31; PE: risk ratio = 1.41, 95% confidence interval: 1.20–1.65) [24]. Additionally, a nationwide US population-based study of 408,253 admissions with compensated cirrhosis, 241,626 admissions with decompensated cirrhosis, and 575,057 admissions without liver diseases demonstrated a significantly higher risk of VTE in cirrhotic patients younger than 45 years (compensated cirrhosis: adjusted odds ratio = 1.23, 95% confidence interval: 1.04–1.46; decompensated cirrhosis: adjusted odds ratio = 1.39, 95% confidence interval: 1.15–1.69) [25].

4. Epidemiology of VTE in liver cirrhosis

The prevalence and incidence of VTE in liver cirrhosis are greatly heterogeneous among studies. Thus, our team systematically reviewed and synthesized the data regarding the epidemiology of VTE in liver cirrhosis [26]. Among the 20 included studies, the pooled incidence and prevalence of VTE in liver cirrhosis were 1% (95% confidence interval: 0.7–1.3%) and 1% (95% confidence interval: 0.7–1.2%), respectively; the pooled incidence and prevalence of DVT in liver cirrhosis were 0.6% (95% confidence interval: 0.4–0.8%) and 0.7% (95% confidence interval: 0.6–0.9%), respectively; the pooled incidence and prevalence of PE in liver cirrhosis were 0.28% (95% confidence interval: 0.13–0.49%) and 0.36% (95% confidence interval: 0.13–0.7%), respectively. Such epidemiological data should be important for physicians and patients to recognize the potential risk of VTE.

5. Risk factors for VTE in liver cirrhosis

Due to the relative rarity of VTE in liver cirrhosis, it is necessary to obtain the knowledge regarding risk factors for VTE and to further screen high-risk patients who will receive medical prophylaxis for VTE. Except for traditional risk factors in the general population (i.e., older age, comorbidity, surgery), which were reported in the second paragraph of this article, two risk factors related to liver diseases have been more widely recognized, such as international normalized ratio (INR) and albumin. First, cirrhotic patients often have an elevated INR, which reflects an auto-anticoagulation status. Thus, it appeared to be reasonable that the risk of VTE would be lower if INR was higher. However, this was not the case. Northup et al. for the first time found that the risk of VTE was not associated with INR [27]. Dabbagh et al. also confirmed that an elevated INR did not protect against the development of VTE during hospitalization [28]. Smith et al. showed that the risk of in-hospital VTE was similar between patients with INR <2.0 and INR ≥ 2.0 [29]. Indeed, our team observed a positive relationship between INR and risk of VTE [30]. This phenomenon should be explained by the fact that INR is a component of Child-Pugh score and reflects the severity of liver dysfunction, rather than the absolute hemostasis disturbance. Second, several studies coherently found a lower albumin in cirrhotic patients with VTE than those without [27, 31–33]. But a statistical significance was achieved in only two of them [27, 33]. Taken together, a prediction algorithm of VTE in liver cirrhosis should be warranted.

6. Prognosis of liver cirrhosis and VTE

6.1. Effect of VTE on the survival in cirrhotic patients

By analyzing the data from the Nationwide Inpatient Sample (1998–2006), Wu et al. found that the in-hospital mortality of compensated cirrhosis was 16.8 and 7.6% in patients with and without VTE, respectively (odds ratio = 2.16, 95% confidence interval: 1.96–2.38); the in-hospital mortality of decompensated cirrhosis was 18.6 and 11.1% in patients with and without VTE, respectively (odds ratio = 1.66, 95% confidence interval: 1.47–1.87) [25]. More recently, a single-center retrospective study of 2006 admissions with cirrhosis by our team also demonstrated an approximately 10-fold higher in-hospital mortality in patients with VTE than those without VTE (33.3 vs. 3.4%, $P < 0.001$) [30].

6.2. Effect of liver cirrhosis on the survival in VTE patients

A nationwide Danish cohort study of 4392 VTE patients, which included 745 and 3647patients with and without cirrhosis, respectively, explored the effect of cirrhosis on the 30-day death [34]. According to the sites of VTE, the 30-day mortality was 7% (95% confidence interval: 5–10%) and 3% (95% confidence interval: 2–3%) in DVT patients with cirrhosis and without liver cirrhosis, respectively; the 30-day mortality was 35% (95% confidence interval: 29–42%) and 16% (95% confidence interval: 14–19%) in PE patients with cirrhosis and without liver cirrhosis, respectively.

6.3. Effect of liver cirrhosis on the development of cancer in VTE patients

A population-based Danish cohort study of 2755 VTE patients with liver diseases, which included 1867 VTE patients with non-cirrhotic liver diseases and 888 VTE patients with liver cirrhosis, explored the effect of cirrhosis of the development of cancer [35]. VTE patients with liver cirrhosis had a significantly higher 1-year risk of cancer than VTE patients with non-cirrhotic liver diseases (4.3 vs. 2.7%).

7. Conclusions

Physicians should recognize that cirrhotic patients are at a risk of VTE. Once VTE is diagnosed, the outcomes of cirrhotic patients would be worse. INR and albumin should be potential risk factors of VTE in cirrhosis. However, until now, no prediction model for VTE in such patients was well established.

Author details

Xingshun Qi[1]* and Andrea Mancuso[2,3]

*Address all correspondence to: xingshunqi@126.com

1 Department of Gastroenterology, General Hospital of Shenyang Military Area, Shenyang, China

2 Department of Internal Medicine, ARNAS Civico, Palermo, Italy

3 Hepatology and Gastroenterology, Niguarda Ca' Granda Hospital, Milan, Italy

References

[1] Ruppert A, Steinle T, Lees M. Economic burden of venous thromboembolism: a systematic review. J Med Econ. 2011; **14**(1): 65-74.

[2] White RH. The epidemiology of venous thromboembolism. Circulation. 2003; **107**(23 Suppl 1): I4-8.

[3] Silverstein MD, Heit JA, Mohr DN, Petterson TM, O'Fallon WM, Melton LJ, 3rd. Trends in the incidence of deep vein thrombosis and pulmonary embolism: a 25-year population-based study. Arch Intern Med. 1998; **158**(6): 585-93.

[4] Oger E. Incidence of venous thromboembolism: a community-based study in Western France. EPI-GETBP Study Group. Groupe d'Etude de la Thrombose de Bretagne Occidentale. Thromb Haemost. 2000; **83**(5): 657-60.

[5] Delluc A, Tromeur C, Le Ven F, Gouillou M, Paleiron N, Bressollette L, et al. Current incidence of venous thromboembolism and comparison with 1998: a community-based study in Western France. Thromb Haemost. 2016; **116**(5): 967-74.

[6] Ho WK, Hankey GJ, Eikelboom JW. The incidence of venous thromboembolism: a prospective, community-based study in Perth, Western Australia. Med J Aust. 2008; **189**(3): 144-7.

[7] Lindblad B, Sternby NH, Bergqvist D. Incidence of venous thromboembolism verified by necropsy over 30 years. BMJ. 1991; **302**(6778): 709-11.

[8] Heit JA, Silverstein MD, Mohr DN, Petterson TM, O'Fallon WM, Melton LJ, 3rd. Predictors of survival after deep vein thrombosis and pulmonary embolism: a population-based, cohort study. Arch Intern Med. 1999; **159**(5): 445-53.

[9] Alikhan R, Peters F, Wilmott R, Cohen AT. Fatal pulmonary embolism in hospitalised patients: a necropsy review. J Clin Pathol. 2004; **57**(12): 1254-7.

[10] Cohen AT, Agnelli G, Anderson FA, Arcelus JI, Bergqvist D, Brecht JG, et al. Venous thromboembolism (VTE) in Europe. The number of VTE events and associated morbidity and mortality. Thromb Haemost. 2007; **98**(4): 756-64.

[11] White RH. Identifying risk factors for venous thromboembolism. Circulation. 2012; **125**(17): 2051-3.

[12] Geerts WH, Pineo GF, Heit JA, Bergqvist D, Lassen MR, Colwell CW, et al. Prevention of venous thromboembolism: the Seventh ACCP Conference on Antithrombotic and Thrombolytic Therapy. Chest. 2004; **126**(3 Suppl): 338S–400S.

[13] Chandra D, Parisini E, Mozaffarian D. Meta-analysis: travel and risk for venous thromboembolism. Ann Intern Med. 2009; **151**(3): 180-90.

[14] Hippisley-Cox J, Coupland C. Development and validation of risk prediction algorithm (QThrombosis) to estimate future risk of venous thromboembolism: prospective cohort study. BMJ. 2011; **343**: d4656.

[15] Rogers MA, Levine DA, Blumberg N, Flanders SA, Chopra V, Langa KM. Triggers of hospitalization for venous thromboembolism. Circulation. 2012; **125**(17): 2092-9.

[16] Tsai J, Grant AM, Beckman MG, Grosse SD, Yusuf HR, Richardson LC. Determinants of venous thromboembolism among hospitalizations of US adults: a multilevel analysis. PLoS One. 2015; **10**(4): e0123842.

[17] Murray CJ, Lopez AD. Measuring the global burden of disease. N Engl J Med. 2013; **369**(5): 448-57.

[18] Global, regional, and national age-sex specific all-cause and cause-specific mortality for 240 causes of death, 1990-2013: a systematic analysis for the Global Burden of Disease Study 2013. Lancet. 2015; **385**(9963): 117-71.

[19] Schuppan D, Afdhal NH. Liver cirrhosis. Lancet. 2008; **371**: 838-51.

[20] Tsochatzis EA, Bosch J, Burroughs AK. Liver cirrhosis. Lancet. 2014; **383**(9930): 1749-61.

[21] Ge PS, Runyon BA. Treatment of Patients with Cirrhosis. N Engl J Med. 2016; **375**(8): 767-77.

[22] D'Amico G, Garcia-Tsao G, Pagliaro L. Natural history and prognostic indicators of survival in cirrhosis: A systematic review of 118 studies. J Hepatol. 2006; **44**: 217-31.

[23] Tripodi A, Mannucci PM. The coagulopathy of chronic liver disease. N Engl J Med. 2011; **365**(2): 147-56.

[24] Sogaard KK, Horvath-Puho E, Gronbaek H, Jepsen P, Vilstrup H, Sorensen HT. Risk of venous thromboembolism in patients with liver disease: a nationwide population-based case–control study. Am J Gastroenterol. 2009; **104**(1): 96-101.

[25] Wu H, Nguyen GC. Liver cirrhosis is associated with venous thromboembolism among hospitalized patients in a nationwide US study. Clin Gastroenterol Hepatol. 2010; **8**(9): 800-5.

[26] Qi X, Ren W, Guo X, Fan D. Epidemiology of venous thromboembolism in patients with liver diseases: a systematic review and meta-analysis. Intern Emerg Med. 2015; **10**(2): 205-17.

[27] Northup PG, McMahon MM, Ruhl AP, Altschuler SE, Volk-Bednarz A, Caldwell SH, et al. Coagulopathy does not fully protect hospitalized cirrhosis patients from peripheral venous thromboembolism. Am J Gastroenterol. 2006; **101**(7): 1524-8; quiz 680.

[28] Dabbagh O, Oza A, Prakash S, Sunna R, Saettele TM. Coagulopathy does not protect against venous thromboembolism in hospitalized patients with chronic liver disease. Chest. 2010; **137**(5): 1145-9.

[29] Smith CB, Hurdle AC, Kemp LO, Sands C, Twilla JD. Evaluation of venous thromboembolism prophylaxis in patients with chronic liver disease. J Hosp Med. 2013; **8**(10): 569-73.

[30] Zhang X, Qi X, De Stefano V, Hou F, Ning Z, Zhao J, et al. Epidemiology, risk factors, and in-hospital mortality of venous thromboembolism in liver cirrhosis: a single-center retrospective observational study. Med Sci Monit. 2016; **22**: 969-76.

[31] Lesmana CR, Inggriani S, Cahyadinata L, Lesmana LA. Deep vein thrombosis in patients with advanced liver cirrhosis: a rare condition? Hepatol Int. 2010; **4**(1): 433-8.

[32] Barclay SM, Jeffres MN, Nguyen K, Nguyen T. Evaluation of pharmacologic prophylaxis for venous thromboembolism in patients with chronic liver disease. Pharmacotherapy. 2013; **33**(4): 375-82.

[33] Walsh KA, Lewis DA, Clifford TM, Hundley JC, Gokun Y, Angulo P, et al. Risk factors for venous thromboembolism in patients with chronic liver disease. Ann Pharmacother. 2013; **47**(3): 333-9.

[34] Sogaard KK, Horvath-Puho E, Montomoli J, Vilstrup H, Sorensen HT. Cirrhosis is associated with an increased 30-day mortality after venous thromboembolism. Clin Transl Gastroenterol. 2015; **6**: e97.

[35] Montomoli J, Erichsen R, Sogaard KK, Kormendine Farkas D, Bloch Munster AM, Sorensen HT. Venous thromboembolism and subsequent risk of cancer in patients with liver disease: a population-based cohort study. BMJ Open Gastroenterol. 2015; **2**(1): e000043.

Chapter 7

Fat Embolism in Orthopedic Surgery

Ismet Gavrankapetanović, Adnan Papović,
Mehmed Jamakosmanović, Elvir Baždar and
Lejla Tafro

Additional information is available at the end of the chapter

http://dx.doi.org/10.5772/67710

Abstract

Every long bone fracture in orthopedic surgery represents a possible scenario for development of embolism complication, especially the fat embolism. There is no scientific explanation why fat embolism occurs and what are the hypotheses for development of fat embolism or the proper way of prevention, but just speculations and possible theories in the evolution of the clinical picture of fat embolism syndrome. Throughout this chapter, the authors will explain the possible theories of development of fat embolism, risk factors, pathology, and pathophysiology during progress of the clinical picture and signs of the fat embolism syndrome and therapy.

Keywords: fat embolism, orthopedic surgery, complications, fractures

1. Introduction

Every long bone fracture in orthopedic surgery represents a possible scenario for development of embolism complication, especially the fat embolism.

2. History

In 1861, fat embolism was first described by Zenker after a railroad accident and a worker who sustained crush syndrome injuries [1]. At the time when it was first described, it was believed that fat from the bone marrow, after a long bone fracture, embolized in the lungs causing pulmonary deficiency. On the other hand, Fenger and Salisbury believed that fat embolized from fractures to the brain causing death [2]. Von Bergmann first clinically diagnosed fat embolism in a patient with a fractured femur in 1873 [3]. Fat embolism was thoroughly monitored and described during World Wars I and II. It was noted by Wong and his colleagues that patients with long bone fractures had a couple of desaturation episodes during the day with prolonged period of total desaturation [4].

3. Pathophysiology of fat embolism

The pathophysiologic mechanism of fat embolism is comprised of two theories—mechanical obstruction and biochemical injury. After a long bone fracture, fat emboli together with erythrocytes and thrombocytes can occlude pulmonary or brain blood vessels. The release of free fatty acids from fat causes local toxic effect on the endothelium, while the activation of platelets and granulocytes causes vascular incident.

Mechanical obstruction of the pulmonary blood vessels occurs because of the size of the embolized particles. In a dog model, Teng and colleagues found 80% of fat droplets to be between 20 and 40 μm, while vessels in the lungs that are smaller than 20 μm become obstructed [5]. Fat globules of 10–40 μm have been found after human trauma [6].

The biochemical theory suggests that mediators from the fracture site alter lipid solubility, causing coalescence, because normal chylomicrons are smaller than 1 μm. Many of the emboli have a histological composition consisting of a fatty center with platelets and fibrin adhered [7]. Large amounts of thromboplastin are liberated with the release of the bone marrow, leading to the activation of the coagulation cascade.

Peltier hypothesized that elevated serum lipase levels present after the embolization of neutral fat hydrolyzes this neutral fat to free fatty acids and causes local endothelial damage in the lungs and other tissues, resulting in FES [8]. This chemical phase might in part explain the latency period seen between the arrival of embolic fat and more severe lung dysfunction. Elevated serum lipase levels have been reported in association with clinically fatal FES [9, 10].

Mudd and colleagues did not find any myeloid tissue in any of the lungs at autopsy in patients with FES and suggested that the soft tissue injury, rather than fractures, was the primary cause of FES [11].

4. Incidence

The incidence of fat embolism is still not completely known. From the studies done on this topic so far, it happens in younger patients more often with lower limb fractures. Its incidence rises with the number of fractured long bones and severity of suffered injuries. Chan and associates found an incidence of 8.75% of overt FES in all fracture patients, with a mortality rate of 2.5% [12]. The incidence rose to 35% in patients with multiple fractures. Other investigators reported the incidence of FES between 0.9 and 3.5% in patients with long bone fractures [13–15].

5. Clinical presentation

Clinical presentation of the fat embolism syndrome starts with hypoxia, abnormalities in the neurological status, as well as development of petechiae that can be found in the region of the head, neck, and chest. Characteristic for development of petechiae is that they cannot be found in all patients, and some studies have shown their presentation in only 20–50% of cases. Also it is important to emphasize fever that follows the clinical presentation from the beginning. For the survival and adequate care of the patient, it is extremely important to recognize the development of fat embolism syndrome at the beginning. It is known that the development of this syndrome starts 1–2 days after the trauma in a period that can be referred to as a latent period. In some studies, the authors have concluded that fat embolism syndrome develops in the first 24 h (in around 60% of all cases), while in the rest of the traumatized patients, it can be recognized in the first 72 h.

For the proper understanding and better and faster diagnosis of fat embolism syndrome, Gurd and Wilson have developed a classification of the symptoms, where they have divided all symptoms in major or minor signs [16]. For diagnosing a fat embolism syndrome, it is necessary to notice one major and four minor signs that are shown in **Table 1**.

Nowadays, some authors in their studies have noticed the rigidity of the criteria mentioned above. In the study done by Lindeque and colleagues, development of the fat embolism syndrome was noticed with following signs: (1) pCO_2 of more than 55 mg Hg or pH of less than 7.3, (2) sustained respiratory rate of more than 35 breaths/min, and (3) dyspnea, tachycardia, and anxiety which they have suggested to be added in the criteria of Gurd and Wilson [17].

5.1. Major signs of FES

Hypoxia – even though pulmonary symptoms can be developed in a traumatized patient by the pulmonary embolism, heart failure, aspiration, or medication reaction, when none of the mentioned pathogenesis can be connected with patient's clinical presentation, fat embolism syndrome must be suspected in differential diagnosis. For a patient, it is very important to be on an oxygen support from the time of admittance in a hospital.

Major signs	Minor signs
Hypoxemia	Tachycardia
Depression of the central nervous system	Fever
Petechiae	Fat in urine
	Fat in sputum
	Retinal emboli
	Decreased hematocrit
	Thrombocytopenia

Table 1. Major and minor signs of fat embolism syndrome.

Neurological status – in order to be monitored on a proper way, a full neurological status must be examined from the time of admittance of a patient. Every deviation in neurological status must be a suspicion on the development of FES. By the studies published so far on this topic, it is noted that in around 80% of patients with FES, some alterations in neurological status have been noticed. It is also of great importance to exclude the factors that can lead to changes in neurological status and that are not connected with FES (hypoxia, head trauma, etc.). Alterations of consciousness or seizures are considered as a bad prognostic sign.

Petechiae – as mentioned before, not all patients with developed fat embolism syndrome have petechiae as a major sign. They are presented in 20–50% of patients with FES, and their distribution can affect not only the head, neck, and anterior aspect of chest but also the axillar region, palate, and conjunctivae and are caused by embolic fat.

6. Treatment options and prevention

There is no strict protocol regarding possible prevention of fat embolism syndrome. It is considered that immobilization of long bone fracture, fast transport to the hospital unit, and immediate stabilization of the fracture can be ways to prevent the development of fat embolism syndrome. Also, fluid compensation and oxygen support from the moment of admittance into the hospital also reduce the risk of development of FES. It is known that oxygen support has value in prevention of FES.

In order to properly follow up the patient's condition regarding development of FES, it is recommended to daily monitor blood pressure, complete blood count, blood gas values, diuresis, and arterial oxygen on room air together with daily clinical examination.

From the moment of admittance into the hospital, increased fluid compensation (saline, Ringer solution, or hypertonic glucose) and low-molecular-weight heparin or acetylsalicylic acid are measures that possibly prevent the development of fat embolism syndrome [18].

Some studies have shown efficiency in preventing FES by giving large doses of corticosteroids immediately after the injury.

Author details

Ismet Gavrankapetanović[1]*, Adnan Papović[1], Mehmed Jamakosmanović[1], Elvir Baždar[1] and Lejla Tafro[2]

*Address all correspondence to: ismetcap@ortotrauma.com.ba

1 Clinic for Orthopedics and Traumatology, University Clinical Center Sarajevo, Sarajevo, Bosnia and Herzegovina

2 Clinic for Anesthesiology, University Clinical Center Sarajevo, Sarajevo, Bosnia and Herzegovina

References

[1] Zenker FA: Beitrage zur Anatomie und Physiologie de Lunge J. Braunsdorf Dresden, Germany; 1861.

[2] Fenger C, Salisbury JH: Diffuse multiple capillary fat embolism in the lungs and brain is a fatal complication in common fractures: illustrated by a case. Chicago Mod J Examin 1879; 39: pp. 587-595.

[3] Von Bergmann E: Ein fall tödlicher Fettembolie. Berl Klin Wochenschr 1873; 10: p. 385.

[4] Wong MW, Tsui HF, Yung SH, et al.: Continuous pulse oximeter monitoring for inapparent hypoxemia after long bone fractures. J Trauma 2004; 56: pp. 356-362.

[5] Teng QS, Li G, Zhang BX: Experimental study of early diagnosis and treatment of fat embolism syndrome. J Orthop Trauma 1995; 9: pp. 183-189.

[6] Levy D: The fat embolism syndrome: a review. Clin Orthop Relat Res 1990; 261: pp. 281-286.

[7] Wozasek E, Simon P, Redl H: Intramedullary pressure changes and fat intravasation during intramedullary nailing: an experimental study in sheep. J Trauma 1994; 36: pp. 202-207.

[8] Peltier LF: Fat embolism: the amount of fat in human long bones. Surgery 1956; 40: p. 657.

[9] Riseborough EJ, Herndon JH: Alterations in pulmonary function, coagulation and fat metabolism in patients with fractures of the lower limbs. Clin Orthop Relat Res 1976; 115: p. 248.

[10] Schuttemeyer W: Klinische auswertungen der lipasebestimmungen zur diagnose der fettembolie. Arch Klin Chir 1951; 270: p. 50.

[11] Mudd KL, Hunt A, Matherly RC, et al.: Analysis of pulmonary fat embolism in blunt force fatalities. J Trauma 2000; 48: pp. 711-715.

[12] Chan K, Tham KT, Chiu HS, et al.: Post-traumatic fat embolism: its clinical and subclinical presentations. J Trauma 1984; 24: pp. 45-49.

[13] Magerl F, Tscherne H: Diagnose, therapie und prophylaxe der fettembolic. Langenbecks Arch Klin Chir 1966; 314: p. 292.

[14] Peltier LF, Collins JA, Evarts CM, et al.: Fat embolism. Arch Surg 1974; 109: pp. 12-16.

[15] ten Duis HJ, Nijsten MWN, Klasen HJ, et al.: Fat embolism in patients with an isolated fracture of the femoral shaft. J Trauma 1988; 28: pp. 383-390.

[16] Gurd AR, Wilson RI: The fat embolism syndrome. J Bone Joint Surg Br 1974; 56: pp. 408-416.

[17] Lindeque BGP, Schoeman HS, Dommisse GF, et al.: Fat embolism and the fat embolism syndrome: a double-blind therapeutic study. J Bone Joint Surg Br 1987; 69: pp. 128-131.

[18] Roberts CS, Seligson D, Hartley B: Diagnosis and treatment of complications. In: Skeletal Trauma: Basic Science, Management and Reconstruction. 5th ed. Saunders; 2015. pp. 579-608.

Chapter 8

Air Embolism

Bojan Biocina, Mate Petricevic and Ivica Safradin

Additional information is available at the end of the chapter

http://dx.doi.org/10.5772/intechopen.68649

Abstract

Air embolism is one of the serious causes of morbidity and mortality in medicine and surgery, especially in cardiac surgery. Various medical and surgical procedures have been associated with the risk of air embolism. In the chapter, all procedures and pathologic conditions will be described, paying special attention to the root cause analysis of the events in any given circumstance. Special attention is to be paid to techniques of risk minimization of this serious complication. The chapter will give an in-depth insight to the anatomical, physiological and other preconditions of air embolism, thus helping the reader to implement preventive measures and to increase patient safety

Keywords: embolism, air, gas

1. Introduction

Air embolism is, although uncommon, a potentially catastrophic event that occurs as a consequence of the entry of air into either arteries or veins. Put briefly, air embolism occurs when atmospheric gas is introduced into the systemic vasculature. Here, it would be prudent to clarify that the most appropriate name for this entity would actually be "gas embolism". In most cases, gas embolism is in fact air embolism, although the medical use of other gases such as carbon dioxide, nitrous oxide and nitrogen can also result in the condition [1].

Air embolism in the vasculature is the clinical entity with the great potential for severe morbidity and mortality. Venous air embolism is more prevalent when compared to arterial gas embolism. Even though the etiology of air embolism will be discussed in more detail later on, it is worth to mention that air embolism is actually predominantly an iatrogenic complication of both diagnostic and therapeutic procedures in different medical specialties [1–6].

2. Etiology

As previously mentioned, gas embolism can be either venous or arterial. The most common causes of air embolism are surgery, trauma, vascular interventions and barotrauma from mechanical ventilation and diving [7–10].

Gas embolism most commonly occurs not only in an anterograde venous course, as is most typical, but also may occur via epidural spaces and/or via tissue planes [2]. Medical specialties with documented cases of gas embolism were comprehensively reviewed by Muth et al. [1]. According to the literature, gas embolism may occur in cardiac surgery, cardiology, critical care and pulmonology, diving and hyperbaric medicine, endoscopic and laparoscopic surgery, gastroenterology, nephrology, neurosurgery, obstetrics and gynecology, otolaryngology, orthopedics, urology, vascular surgery, etc. [9–23]. Among these, air embolism occurs more frequently in neurosurgical and otolaryngological procedures when compared to surgical procedures in other specialties. An air embolism incident during neurosurgical procedures ranges from 10 to 80%.

There are numerous surgical or other non-surgical invasive procedures where gas embolism has been reported as a complication: (1) needle biopsy of the lung (bronchoscopic or percutaneous), lung resection [15–17, 24] and radiofrequency ablation of lung cancer [25], (2) arthroscopy and arthroplasty [18, 26], (3) gynecological procedures (hysteroscopy [19, 27, 28], C-section [29]), (4) gastrointestinal procedures (laparoscopy [30], colonoscopy [21], endoscopic retrograde cholangiopancreatography (ERCP) [20]) and (5) cardiac procedures (heart surgeries performed with cardiopulmonary bypass [22], cardiac implantable electronic devices implantation [23, 31], cardiac ablation procedures of cardiac arrhythmias) [32–34]. Gas embolism has also been described in ophthalmological [35] and dental procedures [36]. Mechanisms for gas embolism differ widely among the specialties. For example, in cardiac surgery procedures, possible mechanisms are the entry of air into extracorporeal bypass pump circuit and incomplete removal of air from the heart following weaning from cardiopulmonary bypass [22]. In neurosurgery procedures, the possible mechanism of gas embolism is entry of air through incised veins and calvarial bone, especially during craniotomy with the patient in a sitting position. What remains common for all the surgical procedures is the intraoperative use of hydrogen peroxide which may cause formation of arterial and venous oxygen emboli [1].

Gas embolism may certainly occur when handling intravascular catheters. Gas emboli can occur at the time of catheter insertion, while catheter is in place, or at the time of catheter removal [37]. Handling different types of catheters, be it venous or arterial (i.e., central venous catheters [10, 38], hemodialysis catheters [39, 40], pulmonary artery catheters [41] and angioplasty catheters [42]) may result in gas embolism. When handling intravascular catheters, one should keep in mind the factors that contribute to gas embolism occurrence (fracture or detachment of catheter connections, failure to occlude the needle hub, dysfunction of self-sealing valves in plastic introducer sheaths, the presence of a persistent catheter tract following the catheter removal, deep inspiration during catheter insertion or removal, hypovolemia that reduces central venous pressure and upright positioning of the patient).

3. Detection of gas embolism

In order to diagnose air embolism, a clinician should first set the suspicion and should assess clinical findings. Many cases of gas embolism are subclinical with no adverse outcomes. Usually, even when symptoms are present, they are non-specific, and a high index of clinical suspicion for possible gas embolism is required to prompt investigations and initiate appropriate therapy. A splashing auscultatory sign indicating the presence of gas in cardiac chambers can be auscultated using stethoscope [1]. Doppler ultrasonography is a sensitive and a practical means of detecting intracardiac air [43, 44]. Transesophageal echocardiography remains an even more sensitive and definitive method for detecting intracardiac gas [45].

Transesophageal echocardiography is currently the most sensitive monitoring device for detection of air presence, detecting as little as 0.02 ml/kg of air administered by bolus injection [46, 47]. The major deterrents to transesophageal echocardiography are that it is invasive, is expensive and requires expertise and constant vigilance that may limit its use to just a well-trained cardiac anesthesiologist or cardiologist [2].

Noteworthy, a decrease in the end-tidal carbon dioxide levels, as determined by capnometry, may be suggestive of gas embolism as well.

4. Management

Early diagnosis and treatment before catastrophic cardiovascular collapse are of utmost importance. In general, there are three principle goals in air embolism management: (1) prevention of further air entry, (2) a reduction in the volume of air entrapped and (3) hemodynamic support [2]. In case of gas embolism, clinician should institute high-flow oxygen to maximize patient oxygenation during the period of hemodynamic instability. Nitrous oxide should be discontinued, and the patient should be placed on 100% oxygen. Administration of oxygen is important not only to treat hypoxia and hypoxemia but also to eliminate the gas in the bubbles by establishing a diffusion gradient that favors the egress of gas from bubbles [1, 48]. In certain cases, therapy with catecholamines is required, as well as aggressive cardiopulmonary resuscitation, if needed. Rapid volume expansion is recommended to elevate venous pressure, thus preventing the continued entry of gas into intravascular space. Normovolemia should be achieved to optimize microcirculation. Colloid solutions are preferable to crystalloid solutions for hemodilution as crystalloid solutions may promote cerebral edema.

Hyperbaric oxygen therapy decreases the size of the gas bubble both by rising the ambient pressure and by causing hyperoxia [1]. There is emerging evidence suggesting that all patients with clinical symptoms of arterial gas embolism should receive recompression treatment with hyperbaric oxygen, which is in fact considered the first line treatment of choice for arterial gas embolism [1, 49–51].

As Muth et al. discussed in their paper [1], there is evidence that heparin may be beneficial in the treatment of gas embolism [52]. The possible disadvantage would be the risk of hemorrhage into the infarcted tissue. Whereas the use of corticosteroid therapy remains controversial and to date is not recommended, the lidocaine therapy has been shown to provide cerebral protection during cardiac surgery [53]. Even with lidocaine, the evidence is controversial [1, 54] and further research is needed to shed a light into its neuroprotective role.

In conclusion, gas embolism is a risk associated with different diagnostic and/or therapeutic procedures in virtually all medical specialties [1]. Arterial gas emboli may be particularly dangerous if they occlude cardiac or cerebral vessels [1]. Whereas hyperbaric oxygen remains the first choice of arteria gas emboli treatment, the mainstays of treatment for venous gas embolism are volume expansion, targeting 12 mm of mercury of central venous pressure, the administration of 100% oxygen, often with ventilatory support [1]. Finally, prevention of air embolism and prevention of further entry of gas in cases of present air embolism remain the Cornerstone Treatment in management of patients at risk for such a clinical entity.

Author details

Bojan Biocina[1*], Mate Petricevic[2] and Ivica Safradin[2]

*Address all correspondence to: bbiocina@kbc-zagreb.hr

1 Department of Cardiac Surgery, School of Medicine, University of Zagreb, Zagreb, Croatia

2 Department of Cardiac Surgery, UHC Zagreb, Zagreb, Croatia

References

[1] Muth CM, Shank ES. Gas embolism. The New England Journal of Medicine. 2000;**342**: 476-82

[2] Mirski MA, Lele AV, Fitzsimmons L, Toung TJ. Diagnosis and treatment of vascular air embolism. Anesthesiology. 2007;**106**:164-77

[3] Sviri S, Woods WP, van Heerden PV. Air embolism – A case series and review. Critical Care and Resuscitation: Journal of the Australasian Academy of Critical Care Medicine. 2004;**6**:271-276

[4] van Hulst RA, Klein J, Lachmann B. Gas embolism: Pathophysiology and treatment. Clinical Physiology and Functional Imaging. 2003;**23**:237-246

[5] Muth CM, Shank ES. Cerebral arterial gas embolism: Should we hyperventilate these patients? Intensive Care Medicine. 2004;**30**:742-743

[6] Shank ES, Muth CM. Decompression illness, iatrogenic gas embolism, and carbon monoxide poisoning: The role of hyperbaric oxygen therapy. International Anesthesiology Clinics. 2000;**38**:111-138

http://dx.doi.org/10.5772/intechopen.68649

[7] Dudney TM, Elliott CG. Pulmonary embolism from amniotic fluid, fat, and air. Progress in Cardiovascular Diseases. 1994;**36**:447-474

[8] King MB, Harmon KR. Unusual forms of pulmonary embolism. Clinics in Chest Medicine. 1994;**15**:561-580

[9] Schmitt HJ, Hemmerling TM. Venous air emboli occur during release of positive end-expiratory pressure and repositioning after sitting position surgery. Anesthesia and Analgesia. 2002;**94**:400-403, table of contents

[10] Heckmann JG, Lang CJ, Kindler K, Huk W, Erbguth FJ, Neundorfer B. Neurologic manifestations of cerebral air embolism as a complication of central venous catheterization. Critical Care Medicine. 2000;**28**:1621-1625

[11] Raskin JM, Benjamin E, Iberti TJ. Venous air embolism: Case report and review. The Mount Sinai Journal of Medicine, New York. 1985;**52**:367-370

[12] O'Quin RJ, Lakshminarayan S. Venous air embolism. Archives of Internal Medicine. 1982;**142**:2173-2176

[13] Hybels RL. Venous air embolism in head and neck surgery. The Laryngoscope. 1980;**90**:946-954

[14] Faberowski LW, Black S, Mickle JP. Incidence of venous air embolism during craniectomy for craniosynostosis repair. Anesthesiology. 2000;**92**:20-23

[15] Al-Ali WM, Browne T, Jones R. A case of cranial air embolism after transthoracic lung biopsy. American Journal of Respiratory and Critical Care Medicine 2012;**186**:1193-1195

[16] Ramaswamy R, Narsinh KH, Tuan A, Kinney TB. Systemic air embolism following percutaneous lung biopsy. Seminars in Interventional Radiology. 2014;**31**:375-377

[17] Hemmerling TM, Schmidt J, Bosert C, Klein P. Systemic air embolism during wedge resection of the lung. Anesthesia and Analgesia. 2001;**93**:1135-1136, table of contents

[18] Andersen KH. Air aspirated from the venous system during total hip replacement. Anaesthesia. 1983;**38**:1175-1178

[19] Guillard E, Nancy B, Floch H, Henckes A, Cochard G, Arvieux J, et al. Intracerebral hemorrhage related to systemic gas embolism during hysteroscopy. Undersea & Hyperbaric Medicine: The Journal of the Undersea and Hyperbaric Medical Society, Inc. 2010;**37**:89-93

[20] Chavalitdhamrong D, Donepudi S, Pu L, Draganov PV. Uncommon and rarely reported adverse events of endoscopic retrograde cholangiopancreatography. Journal of Digestive Endoscopy. 2014;**26**:15-22

[21] Sopena-Falco J, Poch-Vall N, Brullet E, Mendez-Reyes H, Martinez-Bauer E, Junquera F, et al. Fatal massive air embolism following diagnostic colonoscopy. Endoscopy 2013;**45 Suppl 2 UCTN**:E91

[22] Schmitz ML, Faulkner SC, Johnson CE, Tucker JL, Imamura M, Greenberg SB, et al. Cardiopulmonary bypass for adults with congenital heart disease: Pitfalls for perfusionists. Perfusion. 2006;**21**:45-53

[23] Xiao PX, Hu ZY, Zhang H, Pan C, Duan BX, Chen SL. Massive pulmonary air embolism during the implantation of pacemaker, case reports and literature analysis. European Review for Medical and Pharmacological Sciences. 2013;**17**:3157-3163

[24] Horan TA, Pinheiro PM, Araujo LM, Santiago FF, Rodrigues MR. Massive gas embolism during pulmonary nodule hook wire localization. The Annals of Thoracic Surgery. 2002;**73**:1647-1649

[25] Hiraki T, Gobara H, Fujiwara H, Ishii H, Tomita K, Uka M, et al. Lung cancer ablation: Complications. Seminars in Interventional Radiology. 2013;**30**:169-175

[26] Peruto CM, Ciccotti MG, Cohen SB. Shoulder arthroscopy positioning: Lateral decubitus versus beach chair. Arthroscopy: The Journal of Arthroscopic & Related Surgery: Official Publication of the Arthroscopy Association of North America and the International Arthroscopy Association. 2009;**25**:891-896

[27] Sherlock S. Paradoxical gas embolism during hysteroscopy. British Journal of Anaesthesia. 2008;**101**:742; author reply 42-3

[28] Grove JJ, Shinaman RC, Drover DR. Noncardiogenic pulmonary edema and venous air embolus as complications of operative hysteroscopy. Journal of Clinical Anesthesia. 2004;**16**:48-50

[29] Cluver C, Novikova N, Hofmeyr GJ, Hall DR. Maternal position during caesarean section for preventing maternal and neonatal complications. The Cochrane Database of Systematic Reviews. 2013:CD007623

[30] Azevedo JL, Azevedo OC, Miyahira SA, Miguel GP, Becker OM Jr, Hypolito OH, et al. Injuries caused by Veress needle insertion for creation of pneumoperitoneum: A systematic literature review. Surgical Endoscopy. 2009;**23**:1428-1432

[31] Bongiorni MG, Di Cori A, Soldati E, Zucchelli G, Segreti L, Solarino G, et al. Iatrogenic risk of permanent pacemaker and defibrillator implantation. Giornale Italiano di Cardiologia. 2009;**10**:395-406

[32] Doblar DD, Hinkle JC, Fay ML, Condon BF. Air embolism associated with pulmonary artery catheter introducer kit. Anesthesiology. 1982;**56**:389-391

[33] Doblar DD, Hinkle JC, Fay ML, Condon BF. Air embolism associated with pulmonary artery catheter introducer kit. Anesthesiology. 1982;**56**:307-309.

[34] Hinkle DA, Raizen DM, McGarvey ML, Liu GT. Cerebral air embolism complicating cardiac ablation procedures. Neurology. 2001;**56**:792-794

[35] Moon YE. Venous air embolism during vitrectomy: A rare but potentially fatal complication. Korean Journal of Anesthesiology. 2014;**67**:297-298

[36] Davies JM, Campbell LA. Fatal air embolism during dental implant surgery: A report of three cases. Canadian Journal of Anesthesia. 1990;**37**:112-121

[37] Roberts S, Johnson M, Davies S. Near-fatal air embolism: Fibrin sheath as the portal of air entry. Southern Medical Journal. 2003;**96**:1036-1038

[38] Laskey AL, Dyer C, Tobias JD. Venous air embolism during home infusion therapy. Pediatrics 2002;**109**:E15

[39] Levy SD, Oren-Grinberg A, McSparron JI. Paradoxical air embolus after removal of a central venous catheter. Annals of the American Thoracic Society. 2016;**13**:1856-1857

[40] Yu AS, Levy E. Paradoxical cerebral air embolism from a hemodialysis catheter. American Journal of Kidney Diseases: The Official Journal of the National Kidney Foundation. 1997;**29**:453-455

[41] Jastremski MS, Chelluri L. Air embolism and cardiac arrest in a patient with a pulmonary artery catheter: A possible association. Resuscitation. 1986;**14**:113-119

[42] Chang C, Dughi J, Shitabata P, Johnson G, Coel M, McNamara JJ. Air embolism and the radial arterial line. Critical Care Medicine 1988;**16**:141-143

[43] Porter JM, Pidgeon C, Cunningham AJ. The sitting position in neurosurgery: A critical appraisal. British Journal of Anaesthesia. 1999;**82**:117-128

[44] Gildenberg PL, O'Brien RP, Britt WJ, Frost EA. The efficacy of Doppler monitoring for the detection of venous air embolism. Journal of Neurosurgery. 1981;**54**:75-78

[45] Mammoto T, Hayashi Y, Ohnishi Y, Kuro M. Incidence of venous and paradoxical air embolism in neurosurgical patients in the sitting position: Detection by transesophageal echocardiography. Acta Anaesthesiologica Scandinavica. 1998;**42**:643-647

[46] Jaffe RA, Siegel LC, Schnittger I, Propst JW, Brock-Utne JG. Epidural air injection assessed by transesophageal echocardiography. Regional Anesthesia. 1995;**20**:152-155

[47] Furuya H, Suzuki T, Okumura F, Kishi Y, Uefuji T. Detection of air embolism by transesophageal echocardiography. Anesthesiology. 1983;**58**:124-129

[48] Van Liew HD, Conkin J, Burkard ME. The oxygen window and decompression bubbles: Estimates and significance. Aviation, Space, and Environmental Medicine. 1993;**64**: 859-865

[49] Ziser A, Adir Y, Lavon H, Shupak A. Hyperbaric oxygen therapy for massive arterial air embolism during cardiac operations. The Journal of Thoracic and Cardiovascular Surgery. 1999;**117**:818-821

[50] Dutka AJ. A review of the pathophysiology and potential application of experimental therapies for cerebral ischemia to the treatment of cerebral arterial gas embolism. Undersea Biomedical Research. 1985;**12**:403-421

[51] Peirce EC, 2nd. Specific therapy for arterial air embolism. The Annals of Thoracic Surgery. 1980;**29**:300-303

[52] Ryu KH, Hindman BJ, Reasoner DK, Dexter F. Heparin reduces neurological impairment after cerebral arterial air embolism in the rabbit. Stroke. 1996;**27**:303-309, discussion 10

[53] Mitchell SJ, Pellett O, Gorman DF. Cerebral protection by lidocaine during cardiac operations. The Annals of Thoracic Surgery. 1999;**67**:1117-1124

[54] Mitchell SJ, Merry AF, Frampton C, Davies E, Grieve D, Mills BP, et al. Cerebral protection by lidocaine during cardiac operations: A follow-up study. The Annals of Thoracic Surgery. 2009;**87**:820-825

Foreign Intravascular Object Embolization and Migration: Bullets, Catheters, Wires, Stents, Filters, and More

Thomas R. Wojda, Stephen D. Dingley,
Samantha Wolfe, W. T. Hillman Terzian,
Peter G. Thomas, Daniel Vazquez,
Joan Sweeney and Stanislaw P. Stawicki

Additional information is available at the end of the chapter

http://dx.doi.org/10.5772/68039

Abstract

Foreign intravascular object embolization (FIOE) is an important, yet underreported occurrence that has been described in a variety of settings, from penetrating trauma to intravascular procedures. In this chapter, the authors will review the most common types of FIOEs, including bullet or "projectile" embolism (BPE), followed by intravascular catheter or wire embolization (ICWE), and conclude with intravascular noncatheter object (e.g., coil, gelatin, stent, and venous filter) migration (INCOM). In addition to detailed topic-based summaries, tables highlighting selected references and case scenarios are also presented to provide the reader with a resource for future research in this clinical area.

Keywords: intravascular emboli, iatrogenic injury, penetrating trauma, bullet injury, coil migration, intravascular device embolization, catheter or wire embolization

1. Introduction

Both traumatic and iatrogenic foreign intravascular object emboli (FIOE) have been described in the literature [1–3]. Traumatic bullet or "projectile" emboli (BPE) are mostly secondary to bullets or bullet fragments [1, 4, 5], with various types of shrapnel contributing to a smaller number of total cases [6]. In general, smaller caliber projectiles such as shot gun pellets are among the most common BPEs [8]. Iatrogenic FIOE are usually due to venous catheter dislodgement and retained guidewire migration [8, 9]. Such intravascular or wire embolization (ICWE) events continue to occur despite increased emphasis on patient safety and adverse event prevention [10]. As increasingly complex endovascular procedures are becoming commonplace, reports of various types of intravascular objects (e.g., stents, coils, gelatin, and filters) migrating or embolizing to anatomically remote sites have been published [11–16]. Collectively, we have included the latter heterogeneous group of events under the umbrella term "intravascular noncatheter object migration" (INCOM).

The treatment of FIOE has evolved significantly over the last two decades, largely due to advances in endovascular therapeutics. Percutaneous intravascular techniques have become the gold standard in most situations, with surgery serving largely as a last-resort rescue option. Clinical management of FIOE is highly individualized and patient specific. Healthcare providers should be aware of major therapeutic options and any potential pitfalls. This chapter reviews FIOEs by type, specific complications, and clinical management. We will also discuss the most commonly encountered types of intravascular FIOEs, including BPEs, ICWEs and INCOMs associated with endovascular procedures.

2. Bullet or projectile embolism

Bullet or "projectile" embolism (BPE, **Figure 1** and **Table 1**) is a rare phenomenon in trauma, with approximately 300 published cases in the literature [17]. The first instance of a traumatic BPE was published by Thomas Davis in 1834, when he reported a case of a wooden fragment that embolized from the venous circulation to the right ventricle in a young boy [5]. A bullet embolism occurs when a small caliber, usually low velocity bullet, penetrates a single vessel wall and remains within the circulation [4]. Thus, the bullet must be of a smaller diameter than that of vessel, as well as of sufficiently low kinetic energy to traverse only one vessel wall and come to rest within the vascular lumen. In this context, shotgun pellets and 22-caliber bullets are the most commonly encountered projectiles [18]. Nearly all of the cases in literature involve bullets 0.38 caliber and smaller, with only one recorded case of a 0.40 caliber bullet embolism [18]. In rare cases, various fragments of shrapnel have been found to embolize as well [6, 19, 20].

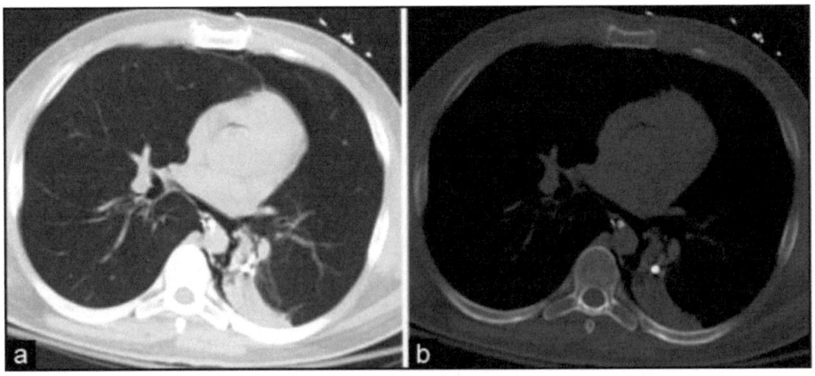

Figure 1. Computed tomography showing a 5 mm bullet that embolized to the left lower lobe pulmonary artery, causing a pulmonary infarction (a = lung window images; b = bone window images). *Source*: Duke et al. [1]. Images used under the terms of the *Creative Commons Attribution-NonCommercial-ShareAlike License (CC BY-NC-SA)*, which permits noncommercial use, distribution, and reproduction in any medium, provided the original work is properly cited.

http://dx.doi.org/10.5772/68039

Author	Patient data	Course of projectile	Type of embolization	Intervention
Carter [4]	22-y/o M shot in the RLQ	Right external iliac vein to the left common iliac vein	Venous	Endovascular
Duke [1]	25-y/o M shot in the left face	Travelled from right jugular vein to the left lower pulmonary artery	Venous	Nonoperative
Huang [32]	19-y/o M, shot in the back	Abdominal aorta at the level of the celiac artery and travelled to the L popliteal artery	Arterial	Endovascular
Koirala [6]	36-y/o M who sustained hammer injury	Patient presented 9 days after a hammer injury left a piece of metal lodged in his R thigh. Following operative exploration of the wound in the Trendelenburg position, the object embolized to his mediastinum, lodging at the SVC-aygos junction	Venous	Sternotomy, with azygous venotomy and projectile retrieval
Lu [22]	20-y/o M shot in the right buttock	Right internal iliac vein to right middle lobe pulmonary artery	Venous	Open, after failure of endovascular
Manganas [20]	39-y/o M presented with massive hemoptysis 30 years after shrapnel blast injury to R chest	Patient sustained a remote shrapnel blast injury as a 9-y/o and presented with massive hemoptysis requiring emergency surgery	Traumatic arteriovenous malformation	Combined intervention; Emergency double lumen endobronchial intubation, arteriography with embolization, and R lower lobectomy
Miller [5]	22-y/o M shot in the left chest	Through the left hemidiaphragm into the external iliac vein, and was found in suprahepatic vena cava	Venous	Endovascular
Miller [5]	52-y/o M shot in midabdomen	IVC above bifurcation of iliac veins, was found in the right ventricle	Venous	Endovascular
Nolan [33]	46-y/o M shot in RUQ abdomen	Infrarenal IVC and travelled to the retrohepatic IVC, retracted into proximal R hepatic vein. It then migrated back to IVC and embolized retrograde to the left common iliac vein	Venous	Endovascular

Author	Patient data	Course of projectile	Type of embolization	Intervention
Padula [28]	32-y/o F who sustained abdominal GSW	Following gunshot wounding in 1952, the patient presented in 1966 with bullet embolism to the heart. Initially (1952) the bullet was lodged in the pelvis, and subsequently became fixated to the annulus of the tricuspid valve. In 1966, she developed acute cough and fevers	Venous	Cardiotomy under cardiopulmonary bypass was performed to retrieve the bullet
Pan [24]	19-y/o M shot in the LLQ of the abdomen	Abdominal aorta and gained access to the IVC through an aorto-caval fistula. It was found in the right ventricle	Paradoxical	Open approach
Ranvier [23]	20-y/o M shot in right buttock	Right internal iliac vein to the right middle lobe pulmonary artery	Venous	Nonoperative, after failure of endovascular
Schroeder [27]	19-y/o M shot in right chest	Right brachiocephalic vein, travelled to the left internal iliac vein	Venous	Endovascular
Stallings [18]	23-y/o M shot in the right shoulder	Bullet travelled from axillary vein to the right ventricle	Venous	Open, after failed endovascular
Yamanari [26]	39-y/o M shot in the left buttock	Left external iliac vein, travelling to the left pulmonary artery	Venous	Nonoperative, after failed endovascular
Yordanov [34]	14-y/o F shot in the right neck	External right jugular vein to superior vena cava to inferior vena cava and into the intrahepatic venous system	Venous	Open approach

Entries listed in alphabetical order, based on first author's name.

Table 1. Summary of selected literature reports involving bullet or projectile embolization.

Several diagnostic findings should prompt suspicion of a BPE. An inconsistent number of entry and exit wounds may be indicative of a retained bullet or projectile. The possibility of an intravascular location of this retained object should be considered when there is no clinical or radiographic evidence of the projectile at any place along the expected course, or if the bullet is found at a distant or inappropriate location based on this trajectory. Additionally, a "migrating projectile" found in different locations on serial or repeat imaging should prompt suspicion of BPE [5].

Most BPEs are arterial (80%) with only 20% being venous [5]. Arterial emboli travel in the direction of blood flow and eventually become lodged in distal vessels, with the potential for resultant end-organ or extremity ischemia and thrombosis [21]. Approximately 80% of arterial emboli are symptomatic due to acute vessel occlusion. Consequently, arterial BPEs are more likely to have early and acute clinical presentation that requires urgent procedural intervention [22]. Surgical BPE removal is considered to be the gold standard, with both open and endovascular techniques described [23].

Venous emboli also generally travel in the direction of blood flow. However, exceptions to this rule do exist. In an estimated 15% of instances, a bullet in the venous system will embolize in retrograde fashion and travel in peripheral direction under the effects of gravity [24]. Even less common, a projectile may become a "paradoxical" embolus if it enters the venous system and subsequently gains access to the arterial circulation through a traumatic arteriovenous fistula or intra-cardiac communication, such as a patent foramen ovale or ventricular septal defect [22]. The incidence of paradoxical emboli was found to be 2.4% in a review by Springer et al. [17].

As previously stated, the vast majority of venous emboli migrate in the direction of blood flow and most commonly come to rest in the pulmonary arterial system or the right heart [17, 25, 26]. A 90-year review of 120 cases of venous missile emboli compiled by Schroder et al. [27] showed that 83% eventually travelled to the right heart or pulmonary artery, and only 4% remained in the peripheral venous system. Significantly delayed venous projectile embolization has also been reported [20, 28].

Clinical consequences of venous BPE migration include pulmonary artery embolism, cardiac valve dysfunction, endocarditis, abscess formation, sepsis, thrombosis, dysrhythmias, intraventricular communications, cardiac conduction defects, tissue erosion, hemorrhage, cardiac ischemia from erosion into coronary vessels, and thrombophlebitis [5]. However, venous emboli are only symptomatic in approximately one-third of the cases, and complications from the initial injury may not occur until months, years, and even decades later [5, 20]. Therefore, treatment of venous emboli has remained controversial.

Symptomatic cases undoubtedly warrant removal, with endovascular techniques being the first line management. The danger of BPE can be exemplified by a case of an abdominal shotgun wound where pellet embolization resulted in bilateral lower extremity amputations [7]. The advent and subsequent progress in the area of endovascular interventions resulted in increased procedural safety and greater BPE retrieval success rates, as exemplified in a report from the 1980s describing removal of embolized bullet from the right ventricle [25]. Aside from previously mentioned complications of venous emboli; symptoms such as fever, pericarditis, pleural effusions, arrhythmia, and thrombi seem to favor BPE removal [5]. It has been proposed that objects >5 mm in diameter, irregularly shaped, freely mobile, or only partially embedded within the myocardium should also be considered for extraction [5].

The management of asymptomatic venous emboli is not clearly defined. In asymptomatic cases, the risk of surgical intervention involving the pulmonary artery or right ventricle must be weighed against the risk of delayed embolic or infective complications. Some authors recommend that retrieval of asymptomatic emboli should be considered only if an endovascular technique can be used, as the risks associated with invasive surgery, up to and including median sternotomy or cardiopulmonary bypass may be too high to be considered on an elective basis [5]. Moreover, existing evidence suggests that there is no significant outcome difference between patients managed operatively versus nonoperatively [29, 30]. In terms of nonoperative management approaches, it has been proposed that patients should undergo serial imaging during outpatient follow-up, with consideration of therapeutic anticoagulation and selective use of antibiotic prophylaxis [23, 31]. The treatment of BPE continues to evolve as endovascular techniques increase in popularity and become safer. BPEs are rare but well-documented occurrences in traumatology, and further studies are required to determine the most optimal clinical management strategies.

3. Intravascular catheter or wire embolization (ICWE)

Vascular access catheters are utilized for numerous indications including long-term antibiotic delivery, parenteral nutrition, hemodynamic monitoring, hemodialysis, infusion of chemotherapeutic agents, and administration of other medications [35, 36]. Complications of vascular access include bleeding, thrombosis, infection, pneumothorax, mechanical occlusion, and rarely, catheter dislodgement/fracture with subsequent distal embolization / migration [11, 35–37]. In a study of 1500 patients with implanted venous access devices, 87% patients had no reported complications, with infection occurring in 4.8%, thrombosis in 3.2%, and catheter fracture in 0.2% cases [38]. Other studies have reported catheter fracture rates of up to 4.1% [39–41]. The utilization of intravenous catheters continues to be high. Inherent to this trend is the growing number of mechanical catheter malfunctions. Therefore, it has become increasingly apparent that effective strategies for dealing with complications of mechanical malfunction, including intravascular catheter or wire embolization (ICWE) must be developed.

Early reports of ICWE date back to mid-1950s [42]. Turner and Sommers described the embolism of a polyethylene catheter that passed from the median cubital vein to the right atrium [42]. At autopsy, a large mural thrombus was discovered at the tip of the catheter with associated myocardial necrosis. In the early 1970s, Bernhardt et al. [43] reported on 28 patients with intracardiac ICWE. In that study, mortality rate was approximately 60% [43]. In 1978, Fisher published a collected series of 42 ICWE cases reporting adequate follow-up data, with associated mortality and rate of serious complications attributable to ICWE being 38 and 71%, respectively [44]. Among causes of death were cardiac tamponade secondary to myocardial perforation, thrombotic events, pulmonary embolism, sepsis, and arrhythmias. The authors emphasized the importance of early extraction of the ICWEs [44].

Several hypotheses have been proposed regarding the cause of catheter fracture. In one review of 215 cases, the so-called "pinch-off" syndrome was found to be responsible for nearly 41% of fractures (e.g., structural failures) [45]. It was thought that mechanical stress due to repetitive catheter compression and movement relative to surrounding anatomical structures (e.g., clavicle, first rib, sharp bend at the thoracic inlet, etc.) was an important factor [46]. When this "pinch-off" sign was present, physical fragmentation of the catheter was reported as many as 170–280 days after the initial placement procedure [37]. Other potential causes of fracture included catheter damage during extraction (17.7%), separation of port and catheter (10.7%), proximal or distal catheter fracturing (11.6%), and unknown reason in 19.1% of the patients [45]. It is likely that within the latter subgroup, unintentional catheter injury during placement or manipulation resulted in fragmentation, without the primary event being clearly identified. In another review of 92 cases, the most common fracture site was found to be at the physical junction of the port and catheter (84%) [40]. Other potential causes of fracture and dislocation include improper connection between the port and catheter during implantation [47] and the use of small syringes leading to elevated pressures in the system [48].

When catheters become disconnected or fractured, they may migrate to the vena cava, right atrium, right ventricle, and ultimately the pulmonary artery. Because the majority of known ICWEs are associated with acute or chronic clinical symptoms, there are many potentially undiscovered and asymptomatic ICWE occurrences. In fact, it has been reported that asymptomatic ICWEs may be seen in as many as 24–36% of cases of embolization [40, 45]. Many patients present with nonspecific complaints of increased catheter "flow resistance" during infusion, localized pain or swelling. In a review of 42 previously published cases of ICWE, only two cases (4.8%) presented with chest pain. Thirty-six percent of cases were discovered incidentally and 29% cases had localized swelling or pain [49]. Less commonly, patients experienced cardiac dysrhythmias such as ventricular tachycardia [49, 50].

Management of ICWEs has traditionally relied on surgical or interventional extraction to prevent future risk of morbidity and mortality. Relatively recent data suggest that ICWE-related mortality has declined to <2% and prompted some to call into question the aggressiveness of ICWE retrieval strategies [45]. Indeed, there have been several reports of retained catheters in asymptomatic patients for prolonged periods of time (e.g., 10–20 years after the original device placement) [3, 51]. In one case, a chronically retained ICWE lodged in bilateral pulmonary arteries was managed without procedural extraction [52]. In another report, a retained catheter dilator was present in the right ventricle outflow tract for >20 years without clinical symptoms and was removed electively during a later coronary artery bypass and aortic valve replacement operation [3].

Prior to the emergence of advanced endovascular techniques, surgery was the only means of removing centrally located ICWEs. In the mid-1960s, it was reported that nonsurgical retrieval of ICWE from the right atrium was possible [53]. Percutaneous ICWE removal has now become the preferred technique due to its high rate of success and low rate of complications [54]. Numerous authors have reported successful ICWE retrieval using a variety of endovascular approaches [54–58]. In the majority of such cases, vascular access has been obtained through central veins (e.g., internal jugular, femoral, or subclavian). However, the use of peripheral intravenous access sites for retrieval has now also been reported [59]. In conclusion, if central embolization of a catheter or catheter fragment occurs and retrieval is indicated, removal should be attempted by percutaneous methods. In the event that these methods are unsuccessful, the decision to move forward with surgical removal should not be automatic. Indeed, if the catheter is unlikely to further migrate or its discovery has been purely incidental, observation with or without serial imaging may be a reasonable approach [3]. Summary of literature reports on the topic of ICWE is presented in **Table 2**.

Study	Study type	Embolic source	Comment
Bindraban [54]	Case report	Port-a-cath	Description of "lasso technique" for retrieval of broken, dislocated port-a-cath fragment
Biswas [50]	Case report	Central line	Percutaneous retrieval w/ triple loop snare
Cheng [40]	Case series	TIVAD	92 cases. Retrieval w/ loop snare
Choksy [59]	Case report	TIVAD	Peripheral percutaneous retrieval
Chow [9]	Case series	PICC	11 pediatric cases. Nonsurgical, percutaneous retrieval
Chuang [39]	Case series	TIVAD	23 dislodged catheters. Retrieval w/ pigtail and loop snare
Kalińczuk [58]	Case series	TIVAD, CVC, and Swan-Ganz catheter entanglement	14 cases. Retrieval w/ pigtail and loop snare
Kim [56]	Case report	TIVAD	Percutaneous retrieval w/ pigtail catheter and gooseneck snare
Kock [38]	Case series	TIVAD	1500 patients. 0.2% catheter fracture rate
Nakabayashi [55]	Case report	TIVAD	Percutaneous retrieval w/ pigtail catheter and gooseneck snare
Pande [57]	Case report	PICC	Nonsurgical removal w/ flexible biopsy forceps

Entries listed in alphabetical order, based on first author's name.
TIVAD, totally implantable venous access device; CVC, central venous catheter.

Table 2. Summary of selected literature reports involving intravascular catheter or fragment embolization.

4. Intravascular guidewire migration or embolization

The use of guidewires in medical procedures to obtain safe vascular access began in the 1950s when the Swedish radiologist Sven-Ivar Seldinger introduced the practice of using flexible guidewires to place catheters into vessels [60]. Since then, the Seldinger technique has become the cornerstone of procedures such as angiography, percutaneous thoracostomy tube placement, certain PEG tube models, and lead insertion for artificial pacemakers or automatic implantable cardioverter-defibrillators [61–66].

One specific procedural approach that almost all medical and surgical trainees will encounter and use is the Seldinger technique for the insertion of central venous catheters (CVC) [67]. CVC placement is usually performed for hemodynamic monitoring, vascular access, or specific treatments that require central vein access. Commonly used points of access include the neck (internal jugular vein), chest (subclavian or axillary vein), groin (femoral vein), or arm (as a peripherally inserted central catheter or "PICC line") [35, 36].

Although there are many different types of CVCs available, the insertion process for all of them is similar. Due to limited scope of the current article, the reader is referred to other sources describing typical procedural steps of CVC placement [68, 69]. For the purposes of our discussion, there are two key safety messages: (a) if the catheter is adequately positioned, all lumens of the CVC should allow for the easy aspiration of blood from the vein and the flushing of saline (or heparin) into the vein; and (b) radiographs should be obtained as a final precaution to ensure that the CVC is not anatomically malpositioned, there is no evidence of pneumothorax or postprocedural bleeding, and to document that the guidewire has been removed [68, 69].

In addition to pneumothorax, central venous catheterization is associated with other, well-described risks, including infection, thrombosis, unintentional arterial puncture, malpositioning, nerve damage, bleeding, venous air embolism, and arrhythmias [35, 36]. It is estimated that between 15 and 33% of CVC attempts result in some sort of complication (including failure to place the CVC) [70, 71]. Specific recommendations exist regarding CVC placement and maintenance care to reduce complication rates, with special focus on eliminating catheter-associated infections [72].

One of the most unusual and poorly described complications of CVC placement is guidewire embolization (GWE, **Figure 2**). GWE is an iatrogenic complication estimated to occur roughly at a rate of 1–2 per several thousand CVC insertions [10, 73]. The event occurs when a guidewire migrates through the venous system causing complications such as arrhythmias, vascular injury, thrombosis, or infection. It is the direct result of a guidewire becoming lost during CVC placement by either not removing the guidewire after the procedure or failing to control the guidewire during the procedure [73].

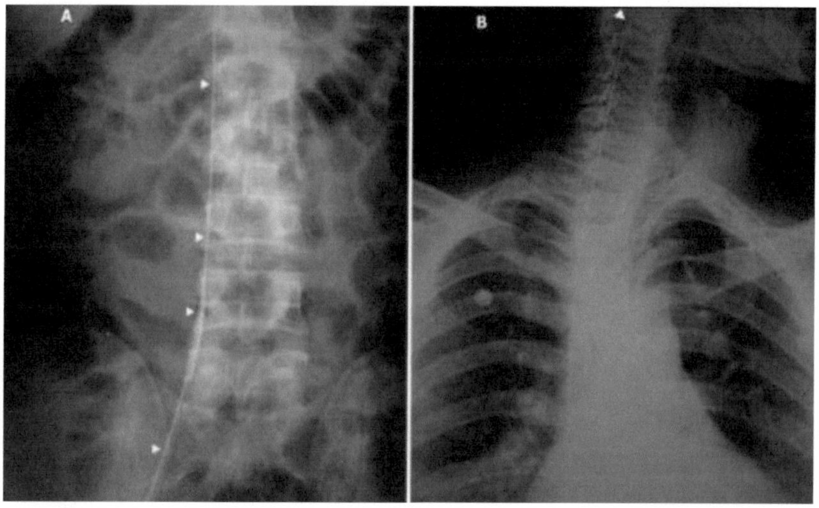

Figure 2. Radiographic images showing a retained guidewire spanning from the abdominal vena cava [A] to the right internal jugular vein [B]. *Source*: Taslimi R et al. [150]. Images used under the terms of the Creative Commons Attribution License (http://creativecommons.org/licenses/by/3.0), which permits unrestricted use, distribution, and reproduction in any medium, provided the original work is properly cited.

Inspect the wire for defects before insertion
If resistance is met during guidewire placement, remove and inspect the guidewire for damage and replace it if needed
Make sure that the guidewire is visible on the proximal and distal ends of the catheter before advancing the catheter
Advance the catheter over the guidewire and do advance the guidewire with the catheter
Hold onto the guidewire at all times until it is removed; if necessary, clamp the end of it while advancing the catheter
Inspect the wire for complete removal at the end of the procedure and document in medical record accordingly

Table 3. Recommendations for decreasing the chances of guidewire loss during CVC placement [77].

While data are lacking regarding the risk of GWE from losing a guidewire *per se*, guidewire loss is the only mechanism for GWE to occur and therefore key technical and procedural safety steps must be followed at all times when placing CVCs [10]. Risk factors for guidewire loss include CVCs placed by inexperienced providers, CVCs placed in emergent situations, operator inattention, inadequate supervision of trainees, and overburdened staff [10, 74–76]. Selected recommendations for decreasing the likelihood of guidewire loss are listed in **Table 3** [77]. All anatomic vascular access points are at risk for guidewire loss and GWE (**Table 4**). It is important to emphasize that GWEs may be discovered at various points in time, sometimes even years after the CVC placement procedure occurred. Listing of selected GWE cases is provided in **Table 4**.

Study	Demographics	Access point	Complications	Resolution	Comments
Ghatak [74]	60-y/o female	Neck—Right internal jugular v.	Guidewire found crossing superior and inferior vena cava junction	Grasped catheter and wire together with forceps and removed both together	Guidewire lost when operator distracted by arrhythmia on monitor
Schummer [77]	63-y/o female	Neck—Right internal jugular v.	Guidewire found within internal jugular v. extending into superior and inferior vena cava	Guidewire removed via right internal jugular v. open surgical exploration	Unsupervised trainee encountered resistance while advancing the guidewire and after placing the catheter, did no know to remove the guidewire. Catheter withdrawn later while guidewire still remained in vein
Schummer [77]	62-y/o male	Neck—Right internal jugular v.	Guidewire found extending from right atrium to right internal jugular v.	Guidewire removed using Dormia basket	Distracted anesthesiologist failed to supervise trainee who never removed guidewire during catheter placement

http://dx.doi.org/10.5772/68039

Study	Demographics	Access point	Complications	Resolution	Comments
Schummer [77]	43-y/o male	Neck—Left internal jugular v.	Guidewire hidden within catheter of left internal jugular v.	Guidewire removed with catheter held in place by two clamps	Found incidentally on X-ray within catheter
Cheddie and Singh [9]	30-y/o male	Chest - Right subclavian v.	Migration to right external iliac v.	Retrieved under fluoroscopy from cannulated right common femoral v. using snare	Inexperienced operator did not hold onto guidewire after inserting it excessively
Ghatak [76]	40-y/o female	Chest – Right subclavian v.	Guidewire found within a pre-existing catheter during hospital admission	Grasped catheter and wire together with forceps and removed both together	Guidewire was never removed after procedure and had been advanced into vein with the catheter
Narendra and Baghavan [80]	64-y/o female	Chest – Right subclavian v.	Guidewire migrated down to right external iliac vein	Removed by open surgical retrieval	Guidewire advanced with catheter by accident
Cheddie and Singh [9]	31-y/o female	Groin - Right femoral v.	Migration to inferior vena cava and superior vena cava, and ultimately into right jugular v.	Retrieved under fluoroscopy through right common femoral v. with snare	Emergent trauma catheter placed where catheter accidentally advanced with guidewire
Schummer [79]	68-y/o male	Groin – Left femoral v.	Guidewire hidden within catheter of left femoral v.	Guidewire removed after catheter removed when it was found to still be sticking outside of skin	Post-procedure X-ray showed wire but it was not reported by radiologist, discovered incidentally when another catheter was placed one day later in a different body vessel
Reynen [54]	53-y/o male	Arm – Right cubital v.	Guidewire found 14 years later with one end at the junction of the left and right pulmonary arteries and the other end in the right ventricle	Guidewire flotation on fluoroscopy was absent. Wire was thought to adhered to vascular wall so extraction not attempted	Diagnosis delayed since patient had concomitant moderate chronic obstructive lung disease

Table 4. Case series of guidewire embolisms arranged by vascular access point.

Whenever there is concern that guidewire loss may have occurred, immediate identification and remedial action is required. As obvious as this occurrence may seem when examining events retrospectively, the fact that GWEs continue to happen suggests that our current approaches are not fail-proof [79, 80]. In this context, commonly reported "red flags" suggesting guidewire loss may include: (a) the guidewire is missing at the end of case and not accounted for; (b) there is resistance to blood aspiration and saline flushing through the distal lumen; and (c) the guidewire is visible on postprocedure radiograph. In the event that guidewire loss occurs and it is not immediately retrievable at bedside, or it is discovered that GWE has occurred, it is recommended that the first basic steps in management is to anticoagulate the patient with intravenous heparin [78] and to initiate intravenous antibiotic therapy [8]. This is usually followed by procedural retrieval of the guidewire. It is critically important to honestly disclose any adverse events to the patient and his/her family.

The need for prompt procedural extraction is supported by the reports that embolic events related to guidewires are associated with complications in 49% of cases and can be fatal in up to 20% of cases [81]. In one unusual case, the guidewire disintegrated and emerged from the patient's neck [82]. Although not strictly a study of lost guidewires, in a series of 220 ICWEs, morbidity exceeded 70% and mortality approached 40% when a catheter fragment causing embolism was not removed [44]. Not infrequently, GWEs are found incidentally on imaging [83]. With more chronic cases of guidewire retention, the foreign object may become incorporated into the vessel wall. In such circumstance, the risk of extraction may exceed the risk of continued retention, especially if there are no clinical symptoms or other manifestations. If there is any question in that regard, fluoroscopy can be performed to help guide clinical decision making. If the retained guidewire fails to exhibit "flotation" within the vessel lumen on fluoroscopy, it has likely become incorporated into the vessel wall [84].

Once the decision to remove a retained guidewire is made, the extraction is preferably performed using percutaneous endovascular techniques. However, if the GWE is in the heart or central vasculature, or if percutaneous extraction fails for any reason, thoracotomy or video-assisted thorascopic surgery may be needed [81]. Devices which have been used successfully in GWE removal (percutaneous and open) include snares, Dormia baskets, bronchoscopy forceps, and surgical hooks [52]. It is critical to remember that as the utilization of endovascular procedures increased over time so did the number of associated complications. **Table 4** provides a detailed overview pertaining to the general area of GWE, including anatomic considerations, retrieval, and morbidity.

5. Foreign object embolization and/or migration during therapeutic procedures

This section of the chapter will discuss the uncommon yet potentially serious occurrence of FIOE associated with therapeutic interventional procedures. Various types of potential FIOEs, event types, clinical manifestations, and management options will be discussed. As previously outlined, we group this heterogeneous group of events under the umbrella term "intravascular noncatheter object migration" (INCOM). Events are categorized by general anatomic location. It is important to note that many of the reports reviewed involve device migration, and that the overlap between "migration" and "embolization" entails certain mechanistic similarities. **Table 5** provides a summary of major clinical events associated with endovascular therapeutic procedures.

Author	Device and location	Comment
Intracranial		
Standard (1994) [85]	Guglielmi detachable coil; anterior inferior cerebellar artery	Dual guidewire technique was used to retrieve the device
Watanabe (1995) [87]	Detachable coil; superior cerebellar artery	Snare type endovascular retrieval device was used during retrieval
Zoarski (1997) [98]	Fibered platinum microcoils; Posterior cerebral artery	Adjustable-size, nonangled microcatheter retrieval device was used
Prestigiacomo (1999) [99]	Guglielmi detachable coil; Posterior inferior cerebellar artery	Goose neck snare "twist" technique was used during retrieval
Raftopoulos (2002) [118]	Guglielmi detachable coil; anterior communicating artery	Minimal transarterial coil hooking procedure used during retrieval
Schutz (2005) [110]	Coil fracture; Siphon internal carotid artery; posterior communicating artery	Loose end of the fractured coil was fixed with a stent at the proximal parent vessel wall
Fiorella (2005) [111]	Stretched platinum coils; superior inferior cerebellar artery, middle cerebral artery	Monorail snare technique was used during the removal of platinum coils; goose neck microsnare
Henkes (2006) [119]	Endovascular coil; basilar bifurcation	Description of coil retrieval using the alligator retrieval device
Vora (2008) [91]	Detachable coil; vertebro-basilar system	Retrieval of displaced detachable coil and intracranial stent described using an L5 Merci device during intracranial aneurysm embolization
O'Hare (2009) [120]	Migrated coil; posterior communicating artery	Description of the use of X6 Merci Retrieval device for removing a migrated coil
Lee (2011) [121]	Displaced/stretched coils; Superior inferior cerebellar artery	Authors describe the use of wire as a snare for "rescue" endovascular recovery of displaced/stretched coils
Leslie-Mazwi (2013) [122]	Displaced coil management; various intracerebral locations	Authors describe the use of stent retriever for removal of displaced microcoils
Nas (2015) [123]	Dislocated coil; internal carotid artery	Description of the use of Solitaire® stent for retrieval of dislocated coil
Cardiovascular		
Chomyn (1991) [124]	Stainless Gianturco coil; right lower lobe pulmonary artery	The authors describe the retrieval of migrated Gianturco coil from the pulmonary artery using flexible intravascular forceps
Sanchez (1992) [125]	Wallstent; right atrium	Authors describe retrieval of a Wallstent misplaced during TIPS procedure using a loop snare
Berder (1993) [11]	Coronary stent; Descending aorta	Authors describe retrieval of a migrated coronary stent from the descending aorta utilizing biopsy forceps and PTCA balloon

Author	Device and location	Comment
Kamalesh (1994) [126]	Inferior vena cava stent; Left pulmonary artery	Authors describe retrieval of embolized inferior vena cava stent from the left pulmonary artery; balloon catheter was used with the aid of trans-esophageal echocardiography
Bartorelli (1995) [127]	Palmaz stent; right atrium	Authors describe transcatheter management of embolized Palmaz stent following superior vena cava stenting
Grosso (1995) [128]	Palmaz stent; left pulmonary artery	Description of the retrieval of dislodged Palmaz stent that occurred during TIPS procedure; the authors utilized an angioplastic balloon catheter with surgical venotomy extraction
Hoyer (1996) [129]	Palmaz stent; Right ventricle	The authors describe transcatheter retrieval of a Palmaz stent embolized from the pulmonary artery to the right ventricle in a child; Retrieval and repositioning procedure is presented
Prahlow (1997) [130]	Wallstent embolization; Right atrium and aorta	Authors describe a fatal complication of TIPS procedure. Embolization of Wallstent led to cardiac perforation with tamponade and death
Feghaly (1998) [2]	Venous stent migration: (a) Left common iliac vein to right ventricle; and (b) Left braciocephalic vein to pulmonary artery	Authors describe endovascular retrieval of two migrated venous stents; balloon catheter-based techniques were utilized; operative extraction from the iliac vein was performed
Marcy (2001) [131]	Strecker stent; right pulmonary artery	Authors describe long-term management of Strecker stent migration from left innominate vein to the right pulmonary artery using anticoagulation and "wait-and-see" approach
Ashar (2002) [132]	Wallstent; Pulmonary artery	Authors describe percutaneous retrieval of a wallstent from the pulmonary artery following migration from the original placement site in the iliac vein; Jugular and femoral approaches are utilized
Abdominal		
Takahashi (2001) [133]	Steel-wire coils; migration from splenic artery to gastric body	Report of steel-wire coil migration into the stomach following arterial embolization of a bleeding splenic artery aneurysm
Ozkan (2002) [134]	Guglielmi detachable coil; erosion from hepatic artery to CBD	Patient developed pancreatitis after erosion of Guglielmi coils into the CBD, 2 years after the original hepatic artery pseudoaneurysm embolization procedure
Turaga (2006) [135]	Embolization coil; Hepatic artery to CBD	Patient developed ascending cholangitis due to coil migration into the CBD; Surgical intervention was required
Dinter et al. (2007) [136]	Embolization coil; stomach	Fatal hematemesis due to coil migration into the stomach and the associated creation of aorto-gastric fistula

Author	Device and location	Comment
Reed (2007) [137]	Embolization coil; aorto-venous fistula involving branch of the renal artery	Embolization coil eroded into the collecting system and passed through patient's urinary tract 1 year after the index procedure
Shah (2007) [138]	Steel-wire coils; migration from splenic artery into the gastrointestinal tract	After migrating from embolized splenic artery pseudoaneurysm, steel-wire coils passed via rectum
Jurałowicz (2010) [139]	Embolization coil; Hepatic artery to common bile duct	Patient developed life-threatening obstructive jaundice after migration of embolization coils from hepatic artery aneurysm to the biliary tree; Endoscopic removal of coils was performed
Miscellaneous		
Cishek (1995) [140]	Coronary artery stent; Dislodgement from coronary balloon catheter to the iliac artery	Authors describe the use of a peripheral angioplasty balloon to withdraw the stent into the arterial sheath and then from the patient
Kiyosue (2004) [141]	Intravascular coils; Coil migration from the ICA to pharynx and the external auditory canal	Radiation necrosis was thought to be contributory to the observed coil migration
Chow (2002) [142]	Embolization coil; migration from internal carotid artery into the middle ear and auditory canal	Management consisted of cutting the coil wire (approximately 25 cm) flush to the tympanic membrane; Patient was doing well at 18 month follow-up
Dagain (2008) [143]	Endovascular coil; Erosion of a coil from ICA aneurysm into the right oculomotor nerve	The patient presented 5 years after the index procedure with progressive diplopia and ptosis; Surgical correction was performed
Choi (2016) [144]	Nitinol clip; Distal migration of the clip with tibial-popliteal artery occlusion	Patient developed critical ischemia of the right lower extremity following StarClose SE device deployment; Surgical embolectomy was performed to correct the problem

CBD, common bile duct; ICA, internal carotid artery.

Table 5. Selected reports of intravascular device/particle migration or embolization; within each anatomic location, reports are arranged alphabetically.

Neurovascular procedures. Endovascular occlusion of intracranial aneurysms is commonly performed; however, coil displacement and migration remains a problem and carries the risk of thromboembolic complications [84]. The reported rates of coil migration (**Figure 3**) range from 2 to 6% [85]. Coils seal the aneurysm from blood flow by inducing thrombosis within the lumen of the aneurysm. Thromboembolic complications represent the greatest risk during the endovascular treatment of an aneurysm, with displaced coil material posing significant additional risks. Protrusion, stretching, fracture or migration of a coil may occlude proximal large-caliber vessels or migrate into smaller distal vessels [86]. Moreover, the coil may migrate with blood flow into smaller-branch vessels or lodge at the bifurcation of a vessel, resulting in limitation of flow and potentially tissue hypoperfusion. Occlusion of either the main artery or distal vessel may result in a variable size territory infarct—a disabling or even fatal event [85].

The risk for coil displacement and migration is influenced by a combination of anatomic and technical factors. Both undersized and/or unstable long coils can result in distal coil migration, especially in wide-neck aneurysms [87]. Tortuous vessels and high flow velocities are thought to increase the potential for coil migration [88, 90]. The use of balloon or stent assistance reduces the risk of coil displacement and migration.

The risk of coil prolapse, in addition to migration, is also a significant concern in endovascular treatment of cerebral aneurysms. When improperly positioned, coils may protrude out of the aneurysm neck, narrowing or occluding the parent artery. Stenting can provide further structural support when placing the coils within a specific location, but also runs the risk associated with additional instrumentation. If the coils do not completely fill the aneurysm, residual blood can enter the neck and cause the aneurysm to refill. Meticulous delivery of coils to avoid catheter tip prolapse and deployment of new coils within a stable coil basket may further minimize the risk for coil displacement [39]. Derdeyn et al. [90], found that aneurysm size and coil protrusion were the most important variables associated with postprocedure ischemic events. Systemic

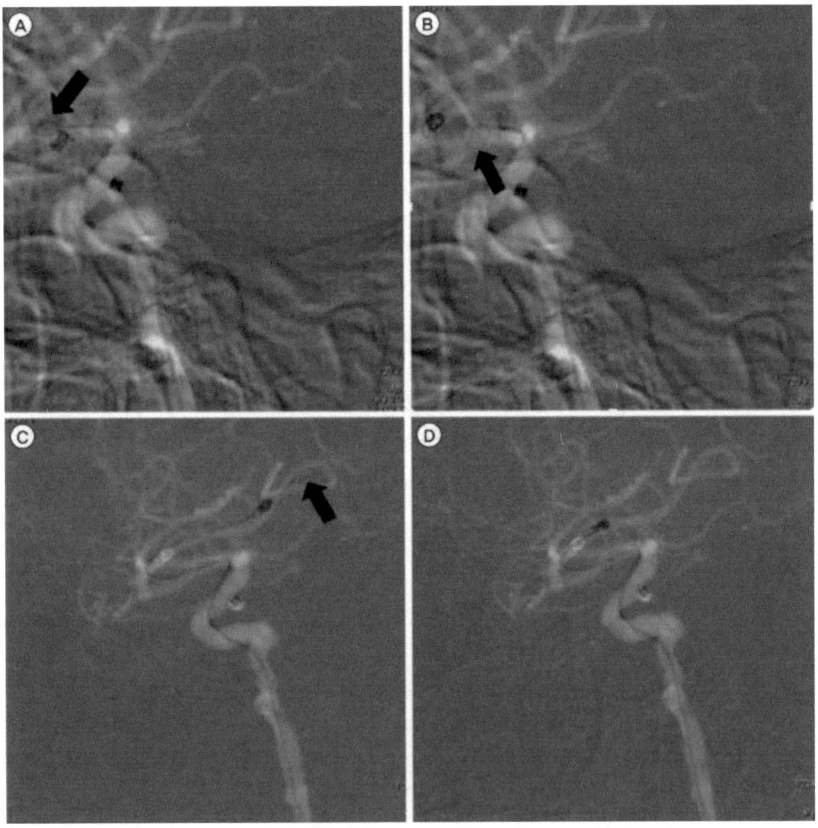

Figure 3. Angiographic images obtained during the coiling of a posterior communicating artery aneurysm. One of the coils migrated into the distal middle cerebral artery (A), requiring the use of a Goose Neck Snare ® (black arrow, A-C) for its retrieval. The right lower image shows the coil being removed after its capture using the snare device (D). *Source*: Oh et al. [151]. Images used under the terms of the Creative Commons Attribution Non-Commercial License (http://creativecommons.org/licenses/by-nc/3.0/) which permits unrestricted noncommercial use, distribution, and reproduction in any medium, provided the original work is properly cited.

heparinization during coil placements may help reduce the risk of thromboembolism; however, definitive treatment is removal of the protruded or migrated coil [89]. Significant coil displacement may necessitate prompt intervention to avoid significant neurological morbidity and mortality [86]. Successful endovascular strategies for retrieval of migrated coils include utilization of wire techniques, snares, retriever devices, and stent retrievers. Microsnares are usually best used during coil retrieval in vessels over 3 mm in diameter, with some risk of vessel dissection or perforation [88, 89]. Among established approaches to coil recovery is the so-called coil stretching with gentle retraction; however, this is only helpful when a coil is not entangled with another device [91]. The L5 Merci Retriever was designed as a device for thrombectomy in the intracranial circulation. However, this particular retriever also carries an indication for foreign body recovery based on trials with earlier models [91, 92]. Intrinsic to the design of the L5 Merci Retriever device is a nontapering helical coil with distally attached arcading suture filaments to ensnare loose particles [91]. These modifications may offer another possible approach for recovery of misplaced coils or stents. Occasionally, endovascular approaches fail and salvage approaches such as microsurgical removal and stent fixation of fractured coil fragments may be employed [86, 93, 94].

Cardiovascular procedures. Indwelling objects, including catheters, wires, and stents may embolize to the heart or the pulmonary artery when utilized in the venous system. Inadequate adhesion to the vessel wall, with subsequent stent dislodgment may be one factor for migration [55]. Within the venous circulation, migrating objects may come to rest at different anatomic levels depending on the location of placement and object size [55, 95]. For venous stents, meticulous procedural planning and selection of the correct device size are both critical. To avoid migration, stent diameter should be optimized to the size and location of the target vein [96, 97]. Stents that migrate from the lower extremities primarily lodge in the right side of the heart and the inferior vena cava, with the superior vena cava and the hepatic veins involved less commonly [98]. In terms of cardiac locations, migrating stents lodge between the inflow area of the right atrium and the inferior atrial or ventricular wall followed by the pulmonary arterial system [99].

Arterial stents may also undergo distal migration [100]. Prevention of such occurrences involves careful procedural planning, including detailed anatomic review of target vessel size and tortuosity [101]. Due to substantial risk of distal complications in such cases, immediate recognition and correction is indicated [102]. Various intravascular and open techniques have been described and successfully utilized to retrieve migrated arterial stents [100, 102, 103]. Operative removal of migrated intravascular stents is associated with high morbidity [104]. For that reason, percutaneous transluminal retrieval must be considered a primary option for the removal of a migrated stent. Exact technique and technical approach depends on stent length and diameter, area of migration, retrieval instruments available, operator experience, and anatomy of the vasculature.

Abdominal procedures. Endovascular interventions have been utilized in a variety of abdominal disease states, from chronic mesenteric ischemia to management of aneurysmal disease [105, 106]. Stent placement for mesenteric ischemia, much like in peripheral vascular disease, can be complicated by distal device migration [107]. Technical considerations are generally similar to those in peripheral vascular disease. Various abdominal aneurysms and pseudoaneurysms have been treated with endovascular embolization, stent insertion, and particle injection [105, 108]. Distal migration of aortic stents, as well as the presence of endoleaks, mandates the use of corrective endovascular techniques [108, 109]. Metallic coils, gelfoam, hydrogel particles, or acrylic glue may be used for embolization [110]. Vascular pseudoaneurysms or aneurysms with a narrow neck benefit greatly from coil embolization and wide-neck, large diameter structures are best treated with a stent [111].

More selective visceral artery embolizations may be also associated with INCOM and significant postprocedural complications. Udd et al. [112] reported a morbidity rate of 17% in a series of embolizations for bleeding pseudoaneurysms due to chronic pancreatitis. In that study, endovascular complications included one localized coil migration requiring procedural retrieval and one distal coil embolization to the iliac artery necessitating operative intervention [112].

Unintended therapeutic particle embolization. Injectable particles used to embolize tumors or to achieve hemostasis in cases of traumatic hemorrhage can unintentionally embolize outside of the intended target area and cause remote end-organ injury [113, 114]. In one case, a stainless steel coil originally placed in the left renal artery migrated into the distal left common femoral artery [113]. In another study, bile duct necrosis occurred at high rates following transcatheter hepatic arterial embolization using Gelfoam powder potentially due to an unintended particle dispersion pattern [115]. Particle INCOM has also been described following intracranial tumor embolization procedures, although the mechanism behind this phenomenon is not fully understood [114]. Finally, Mehta et al. [116], discuss the potential risk of hydrophilic polymer emboli introduced into the vasculature during interventional procedures (e.g., cardiac catheterization, diagnostic, and therapeutic angiography). Associated clinical sequelae may include pulmonary infarct, stroke, and distal hypoperfusion reported days to weeks following suspected INCOM events [116]. In addition to listing cases of intravascular embolization and/or migration of various iatrogenic objects, **Table 5** also includes a number of instances where intravascular devices have migrated and eroded out of the vascular tree.

Complications of particulate foreign body embolization with cerebral angiography have also been described since the 1960s [117]. Shannon et al. [117], reviewed 5 years of autopsies related to postangiogram complications, looking at histological specimens from surgically resected cerebral arteriovenous malformations (AVMs). The results revealed three patients with cerebrovascular events likely related to particulate cotton fiber, gelfoam or polyvinyl alcohol embolization during diagnostic and therapeutic angiography. Possible theories include that the cotton fibers from guazepads, sponges, surgical drapes, etc. carry loosely woven synthetic fibers. These fibers may also be attracted to the glue utilized in AVM repair and travel with the liquid adhesive during the procedure. AVM embolization is typically a much longer procedure than conventional angiography alone, and this greater duration of "at risk" time may help facilitate catheter or guidewire contamination from these extraneous particles. Another comorbid factor includes difficult vascular access due to proximal atherosclerosis in affected patients, as noted during the procedure and by pathology sampling [117].

6. IVC filter migration and embolization

Although relatively rare, intravascular IVC filter migration and filter fragment embolization have been described [145]. Tam et al. [146] reported that the incidence of filter device fracture was relatively high (7.2%) and involved 5.5% of recipients of the Bard Recovery Filter. This incidence rate has been corroborated by others [15]. Certain anatomic factors may lead to the formation of concentrated stress points and thus may cause predisposition for device failure. Specific risk factors include deployment in a tortuous vena cava, deployment over renal ostia, and placement adjacent to a vertebral osteophyte [15]. In descending order, the most common sites for filter fragment embolization were pulmonary arteries (31%), iliac/femoral veins (27%), and the right ventricle and renal vein (3.8% each) [146]. Factors that increase the risk of filter migration and embolization include the so-called "mega-IVC" (e.g., IVC diameter ≥28mm), filter malpositioning, and a large embolus creating a "sail effect" that then dislodges the filter from the IVC, with subsequent embolization to the heart [147–149]. A fracture-free survival model described by Tam et al., predicted a fracture rate of 40% at 5.5 years [146]. In one case, a broken IVC filter strut embolized to the heart, causing cardiac tamponade with hemodynamic collapse approximately 6 years after original placement procedure [149].

7. Conclusions

Foreign body embolism is a relatively heterogeneous grouping of rare but well-known complications. In aggregate, a vast majority of these events are iatrogenic in nature and involve retained catheters, wires, and various types of intravascular particles. Traumatic projectile fragments are well documented but far less common. Depending on the symptomatology, these unusual embolic events may go unnoticed for a period of time and may or may not require surgical intervention. The type and location of the emboli will dictate clinical approaches, with preference for endovascular retrieval with open surgical options reserved for the occasional case of unsuccessful minimally invasive intervention.

Author details

Thomas R. Wojda[1,2], Stephen D. Dingley[1], Samantha Wolfe[1], W. T. Hillman Terzian[1], Peter G. Thomas[2], Daniel Vazquez[3], Joan Sweeney[4] and Stanislaw P. Stawicki[2,5]*

*Address all correspondence to: stawicki.ace@gmail.com

1 Department of Surgery, St. Luke's University Health Network, Bethlehem, Pennsylvania, USA

2 Regional Level I Trauma Center, St. Luke's University Health Network, Bethlehem, Pennsylvania, USA

3 Department of Surgery, The Ohio State University College of Medicine, Columbus, Ohio, USA

4 Center for Neuroscience, St. Luke's University Health Network, Bethlehem, Pennsylvania, USA

5 Department of Research & Innovation, St. Luke's University Health Network, Bethlehem, Pennsylvania, USA

References

[1] Duke, E., A.A. Peterson, and W.K. Erly, Migrating bullet: A case of a bullet embolism to the pulmonary artery with secondary pulmonary infarction after gunshot wound to the left globe. Journal of Emergencies, Trauma, and Shock, 2014. **7**(1): pp. 38-40.

[2] El Feghaly, M., et al., Endovascular retrieval of two migrated venous stents by means of balloon catheters. Journal of Vascular Surgery, 1998. **28**(3): pp. 541-546.

[3] Holley, C.T., et al., Retained catheter dilator in right ventricular outflow tract for 22 years. Journal of Cardiac Surgery, 2013. **28**(6): pp. 679-681.

[4] Carter, C.O., et al., Venous bullet embolism and subsequent endovascular retrieval—A case report and review of the literature. International Journal of Surgery Case Reports, 2012. **3**(12): pp. 581-583.

[5] Miller, K.R., et al., The evolving management of venous bullet emboli: a case series and literature review. Injury, 2011. **42**(5): pp. 441-446.

[6] Koirala, B., et al., Migration of a piece of shrapnel: femoral vein to superior vena cava—azygous junction. European Journal of Cardio-thoracic Surgery, 2012. **42**(3): pp. 584-586.

[7] Sandler, G., et al., Abdominal shotgun wound with pellet embolization leading to bilateral lower limb amputation: case report and review of the literature of missile emboli over the past 10 years. Journal of Trauma and Acute Care Surgery, 2009. **67**(6): pp. E202-208.

[8] Cheddie, S. and B. Sing, Guidewire embolism during central venous catheterization: Options in management. The Internet Journal of Surgery, 2013. **30**: p. 1.

[9] Chow, L.M., et al., Peripherally inserted central catheter (PICC) fracture and embolization in the pediatric population. The Journal of Pediatrics, 2003. **142**(2): pp. 141-144.

[10] Moffatt-Bruce, S.D., et al., Intravascular retained surgical items: a multicenter study of risk factors. Journal of Surgical Research, 2012. **178**(1): pp. 519-523.

[11] Berder, V., et al., Retrieval of a lost coronary stent from the descending aorta using a PTCA balloon and biopsy forceps. Catheterization and Cardiovascular Diagnosis, 1993. **28**(4): pp. 351-353.

[12] Abad, J., et al., Bronchial migration of pulmonary arterial coil. Cardiovascular and Interventional Radiology, 1990. **13**(6): pp. 345-346.

[13] Rosch, J., F.S. Keller, and C.T. Dotter, Materials and methods for transcatheter vascular occlusion: Some personal, practical views. Therapeutic Angiography, 1980, **3**(4): pp. 242-243.

[14] Bach, J.A., et al., Superior vena cava filter. In: Endovascular Interventions. 2014, New York, NY. pp. 1003-1011.

[15] Cipolla, J., et al., Complications of vena cava filters: a comprehensive clinical review. OPUS 12 Scientist, 2008. **2**(2): pp. 11-24.

[16] Stawicki, S.P., et al., Vena cava filters: a synopsis of complications and related topics. The Journal of Vascular Access, 2008. **9**(2): pp. 102-110.

[17] Springer, J., W. Newman, and R. McGoey, Intravascular bullet embolism to the right atrium. Journal of Forensic Sciences, 2011. **56**: S259–S262.

[18] Stallings, L.A., et al., Right ventricular bullet embolism: Diagnostic and therapeutic decisions. Injury Extra, 2013. **44**(7): pp. 64-66.

[19] Andrews, C.M., et al., Venous fragment embolism to the pulmonary artery: A rare occurrence-case report and literature review of venous fragment embolization to the pulmonary artery. Military Medicine Radiology Corner. 2009. **174**. pp. 1-8.

[20] Manganas, C., et al., Traumatic pulmonary arteriovenous malformation presenting with massive hemoptysis 30 years after penetrating chest injury. The Annals of Thoracic Surgery, 2003. **76**(3): pp. 942-944.

[21] Khalifeh, M., et al., Penetrating missile embolisation. European Journal of Vascular Surgery, 1993. **7**(4): pp. 467-469.

[22] Lu, K., et al., Approach to management of intravascular missile emboli: Review of the literature and case report. Western Journal of Emergency Medicine, 2015. **16**(4): p. 489.

[23] Fernandez-Ranvier, G.G., et al., Pulmonary artery bullet embolism—Case report and review. International Journal of Surgery Case Reports, 2013. **4**(5): pp. 521-523.

[24] Pan, G.Z., et al., Bullet embolization from an aorto-caval fistula to the heart. Interactive Cardiovascular and Thoracic Surgery, 2013. **16**(5): pp. 710-711.

[25] Hartzler, G., Percutaneous transvenous removal of a bullet embolus to the right ventricle. The Journal of Thoracic and Cardiovascular Surgery, 1980. **80**(1): p. 153.

[26] Yamanari, M.G., et al., Bullet embolism of pulmonary artery: A case report. Radiologia Brasileira, 2014. **47**(2): pp. 128-130.

[27] Schroeder, M.E., et al., Retrograde migration and endovascular retrieval of a venous bullet embolus. Journal of Vascular Surgery, 2011. **53**(4): pp. 1113-1115.

[28] Padula, R.T., S.C. Sandler, and R. Camishion, Delayed bullet embolization to the heart following abdominal gunshot wound. Annals of Surgery, 1969. **169**(4): p. 599.

[29] Kortbeek, J.B., J.A. Clark, and R.C. Carraway, Conservative management of a pulmonary artery bullet embolism: case report and review of the literature. Journal of Trauma and Acute Care Surgery, 1992. **33**(6): pp. 906-908.

[30] SHANNON, F.L., et al., Venous bullet embolism: rationale for mandatory extraction. Journal of Trauma and Acute Care Surgery, 1987. **27**(10): pp. 1118-1122.

[31] Dato, G.M.A., et al., Posttraumatic and iatrogenic foreign bodies in the heart: report of fourteen cases and review of the literature. The Journal of Thoracic and Cardiovascular Surgery, 2003. **126**(2): pp. 408-414.

[32] Huang, J., et al., Popliteal artery embolism of bullet after abdominal gunshot wound. Radiology Case Reports, 2016. **11**(4): pp. 282-286.

[33] Nolan, T., et al. Bullet embolization: multidisciplinary approach by interventional radiology and surgery. In: Semin intervent Radiol 2012; **29**(03): 192-196. New York, NY: Thieme Medical Publishers.

[34] Yordanov, Y., D. Pateron, and A. May, An unusual aetiology of abdominal pain: the forgotten bullet. BMJ Case Reports, 2014. **2014**: p. bcr2014208268.

[35] Evans, D., et al., Complications associated with pulmonary artery catheters: a comprehensive clinical review. Scandinavian Journal of Surgery, 2009. **98**(4): pp. 199-208.

[36] Kornbau, C., et al., Central line complications. International Journal of Critical Illness and Injury Science, 2015. **5**(3): p. 170.

[37] Damascelli, B., et al., Placement of long-term central venous catheters in outpatients: study of 134 patients over 24,596 catheter days. American Journal of Roentgenology, 1997. **168**(5): pp. 1235-1239.

[38] Kock, H.-J., et al., Implantable vascular access systems: experience in 1500 patients with totally implanted central venous port systems. World Journal of Surgery, 1998. **22**(1): pp. 12-16.

[39] Chuang, M.-T., et al., Concurrent use of pigtail and loop snare catheters for percutaneous retrieval of dislodged central venous port catheter. The Kaohsiung Journal of Medical Sciences, 2011. **27**(11): pp. 514-519.

[40] Cheng, C.-C., et al., Percutaneous retrieval of dislodged totally implantable central venous access system in 92 cases: experience in a single hospital. European Journal of Radiology, 2009. **69**(2): pp. 346-350.

[41] Charvat, J., et al., Implantation of central venous ports with catheter insertion via the right internal jugular vein in oncology patients—single center experience. Supportive Care in Cancer, 2006. **14**(11): pp. 1162-1165.

[42] Turner, D.D. and S.C. Sommers, Accidental passage of a polyethylene catheter from cubital vein to right atrium: report of a fatal case. New England Journal of Medicine, 1954. **251**(18): pp. 744-745.

[43] Bernhardt, L.C., J.T. Mendenhall, and G.P. Wegner, Intravenous catheter embolization to the pulmonary artery. Chest Journal, 1970. **57**(4): pp. 329-332.

[44] Fisher, R.G. and R. Ferreyro, Evaluation of current techniques for nonsurgical removal of intravascular iatrogenic foreign bodies. American Journal of Roentgenology, 1978. **130**(3): pp. 541-548.

[45] Surov, A., et al., Intravascular embolization of venous catheter—causes, clinical signs, and management: a systematic review. Journal of Parenteral and Enteral Nutrition, 2009. **33**(6): pp. 677-685.

[46] Lafreniere, R., Indwelling subclavian catheters and a visit with the "pinched-off sign". Journal of Surgical Oncology, 1991. **47**(4): pp. 261-264.

[47] Ballarini, C., et al., Complications of subcutaneous infusion port in the general oncology population. Oncology, 1999. **56**(2): pp. 97-102.

[48] Lam, A.W.-C., et al., Disconnection of a venous Port-A-Cath followed by embolization after saline flush: rare case report. Japanese Journal of Clinical Oncology, 1999. **29**(12): pp. 643-645.

[49] Denny, M.A. and L.R. Frank, Ventricular tachycardia secondary to Port-a-Cath® fracture and embolization. The Journal of Emergency Medicine, 2003. **24**(1): pp. 29-34.

[50] Biswas, S. and P. McNerney, Ventricular tachycardia from a central line fracture fragment embolus: a rare complication of a commonly used procedure—a case report and review of the relevant literature. Case Reports in Critical Care, 2015. **2015**:265326.

[51] Thanigaraj, S., A. Panneerselvam, and J. Yanos, Retrieval of an IV catheter fragment from the pulmonary artery 11 years after embolization. Chest, 2000. **117**(4): pp. 1209-1211.

[52] Reynen, K., 14-year follow-up of central embolization by a guide wire. New England Journal of Medicine, 1993. **329**(13): pp. 970-971.

[53] THOMAS, J., et al., Nonsurgical retrieval of a broken segment of steel spring guide from the right atrium and inferior vena cava. Circulation, 1964. **30**(1): pp. 106-108.

[54] Bindraban, N.R., et al., Lasso technique for retrieving a broken, dislocated port-a-cath fragment. Netherlands Heart Journal, 2009. **17**(2): pp. 75-6.

[55] Nakabayashi, K., et al., Successful retrieval of a dismembered central venous catheter stuck to the right pulmonary artery using a stepwise approach. Case Reports in Cardiology, 2016. **2016**:6294263.

[56] Kim, O.K., et al., Transluminal removal of a fractured and embolized indwelling central venous catheter in the pulmonary artery. The Korean Journal of Internal Medicine, 2006. **21**(3): pp. 187-190.

[57] Pande, A., et al., Retrieval of embolized intracardiac peripherally inserted central catheter line: novel percutaneous technique by utilizing a flexible biopsy forceps. Heart Views, 2015. **16**(4): p. 154.

[58] Kalińczuk, Ł., et al., Percutaneous retrieval of centrally embolized fragments of central venous access devices or knotted Swan-Ganz catheters. Clinical report of 14 retrievals with detailed angiographic analysis and review of procedural aspects. Advances in Interventional Cardiology, 2016. **12**(2): p. 44.

[59] Choksy, P., S.S. Zaidi, and D. Kapoor, Removal of intracardiac fractured port-A catheter utilizing an existing forearm peripheral intravenous access site in the cath lab. Journal of Invasive Cardiology, 2014. **26**(2): pp. 75-76.

[60] Seldinger, S.I., Catheter replacement of the needle in percutaneous arteriography: a new technique. Acta Radiologica, 1953. **39**(5): pp. 368-376.

[61] Mao, M., et al., Complications of chest tubes: a focused clinical synopsis. Current Opinion in Pulmonary Medicine, 2015. **21**(4): pp. 376-386.

[62] Kwiatt, M., et al., Thoracostomy tubes: A comprehensive review of complications and related topics. International Journal of Critical Illness and Injury Science, 2014. **4**(2): pp. 143-155.

[63] Schrag, S.P., et al., Complications related to percutaneous endoscopic gastrostomy (PEG) tubes. A comprehensive clinical review. Journal of Gastrointestinal Liver Diseases, 2007. **16**(4): pp. 407-418.

[64] Stewart, J.R. and V.L. Gott, The use of a Seldinger wire technique for pericardiocentesis following cardiac surgery. The Annals of Thoracic Surgery, 1983. **35**(4): pp. 467-468.

[65] Luboz, V., et al., ImaGiNe Seldinger: first simulator for Seldinger technique and angiography training. Computer Methods and Programs in Biomedicine, 2013. **111**(2): pp. 419-434.

[66] Boyer, L., et al., Study of the supra-aortic trunks using the humeral Seldinger technique and digitalized angiography of the aortic arch. Apropos of 175 cases. Journal of Radiology, 1991. **72**(10): pp. 497-502.

[67] Macnab, A.J. and M. Macnab, Teaching pediatric procedures: the Vancouver model for instructing Seldinger's technique of central venous access via the femoral vein. Pediatrics, 1999. **103**(1): pp. e8-8.

[68] CliniSnips. Central line placement 2008 January 15, 2017]; Available from: https:// www.youtube.com/watch?v=Lb1Z3bndmA8.

[69] Mubarak, G.S. Subclavian central venous catheterization: Theory & practice. 2013 January 15, 2017]; Available from: https://www.youtube.com/watch?v=RDtgzNWmYBw.

[70] McGee, D.C. and M.K. Gould, Preventing complications of central venous catheterization. New England Journal of Medicine, 2003. **348**(12): pp. 1123-1133.

[71] Eisen, L.A., et al., Mechanical complications of central venous catheters. Journal of Intensive Care Medicine, 2006. **21**(1): pp. 40-46.

[72] O'Grady, N. P., et al., Guidelines for the prevention of intravascular catheter-related infections, 2011. Available online at: https://www.cdc.gov/hicpac/pdf/guidelines/bsi-guidelines-2011.pdf Last accessed on March 29, 2017.

[73] Kusminsky, R.E., Complications of central venous catheterization. Journal of the American College of Surgeons, 2007. **204**(4): pp. 681-696.

[74] Ghatak, T., et al., Accidental guide-wire loss during central venous catheterization: A report of two life-threatening cases. Indian Journal of Critical Care Medicine, 2013. **17**(1): p. 53.

[75] Pokharel, K., et al., Missed central venous guide wires: A systematic analysis of published case reports. Critical Care Medicine, 2015. **43**(8): pp. 1745-1756.

[76] Nadaf, A., et al., Embolization of lost guide wire: mishap or blunder? Medico-legal Update, 2015. **15**(2):127-131.

[77] Schummer, W., et al., Loss of the guide wire: mishap or blunder? British Journal of Anaesthesia, 2002. **88**(1): pp. 144-146.

[78] Narendra, H. and K. Baghavan, Guide-wire embolism during subclavian vein catheterization by Seldinger technique. Indian Journal of Critical Care Medicine, 2006. **10**(4): p. 257.

[79] Arrayhani, M., et al., Unrecognized migration of an entire guide wire during hemodialysis catheter placement. Saudi Journal of Kidney Diseases and Transplantation, 2012. **23**(5): pp. 1059-1059.

[80] Waite, S., et al., Interpretive error in radiology. American Journal of Roentgenology. 2017;**208**: 739-749.

[81] Roye, G., et al., Management of catheter emboli. Southern Medical Journal, 1996. **89**(7): pp. 714-717.

[82] Guo, H., J.D. Lee, and M. Guo, Guidewire loss: mishap or blunder? Heart, 2006. **92**(5): p. 602.

[83] Cassie, C.D., M.S. Ginsberg, and D.M. Panicek, Unsuspected retained 60-cm intravenous guidewire. Clinical Imaging, 2006. **30**(4): pp. 287-290.

[84] Lamprecht, W., Clinical aspects of iatrogenic intracardial foreign bodies. Der Chirurg; Zeitschrift fur alle Gebiete der operativen Medizen, 1965. **36**: pp. 182-183.

[85] Standard, S.C., et al., Retrieval of a Guglielmi detachable coil after unraveling and fracture: case report and experimental results. Neurosurgery, 1994. **35**(5): pp. 994-999.

[86] Ding, D. and K.C. Liu, Management strategies for intraprocedural coil migration during endovascular treatment of intracranial aneurysms. Journal of Neurointerventional Surgery, 2014. **6**(6): pp. 428-431.

[87] WATANABE, A., et al., Retrieval of a migrated detachable coil. Neurologia Medico-Chirurgica, 1995. **35**(4): pp. 247-250.

[88] Henkes, H., et al., A new device for endovascular coil retrieval from intracranial vessels: alligator retrieval device. American Journal of Neuroradiology, 2006. **27**(2): pp. 327-329.

[89] Kung, D.K., et al., Treatment of endovascular coil and stent migration using the merci retriever: report of three cases. Case Reports in Medicine, 2012. **2012**:242101.

[90] Derdeyn, C.P., et al., Postprocedure ischemic events after treatment of intracranial aneurysms with Guglielmi detachable coils. Journal Neurosurgery, 2002. **96**(5): pp. 837-843.

[91] Vora, N., et al., Retrieval of a displaced detachable coil and intracranial stent with an L5 Merci Retriever during endovascular embolization of an intracranial aneurysm. Journal of Neuroimaging, 2008. **18**(1): pp. 81-84.

[92] Felten, R.P., et al., The Food and Drug Administration medical device review process: clearance of a clot retriever for use in ischemic stroke. Stroke, 2005. **36**(2): pp. 404-406.

[93] Rodriguez, G.J., A. Maud, and M.H. Qureshi, Complications in endovascular embolization of intracranial aneurysms: prevention and bailout techniques. In: Complications of Neuroendovascular Procedures and Bailout Techniques (Khatri R, Rodriguez GJ, Raymond J, and Qureshi AI, Eds), Cambridge University Press, Cambridge, UK, 2016: pp. 10-43.

[94] Ding, D., R.M. Starke, and K.C. Liu, Microsurgical strategies following failed endovascular treatment with the pipeline embolization device: case of a giant posterior cerebral artery aneurysm. Journal of Cerebrovascular and Endovascular Neurosurgery, 2014. **16**(1): pp. 26-31.

[95] Kwak, H.-S., et al., Stents in common iliac vein obstruction with acute ipsilateral deep venous thrombosis: early and late results. Journal of Vascular and Interventional Radiology, 2005.**16**(6): http://www.sciencedirect.com/science/article/pii/S1051044307606861.

[96] Raju, S., P. Tackett, and P. Neglen, Reinterventions for nonocclusive iliofemoral venous stent malfunctions. Journal of Vascular Surgery, 2009. **49**(2): pp. 511-518.

[97] Antonucci, F., et al., Placement of venous stents: clinical experience with a self-expanding prosthesis. Radiology, 1992. **183**(2): pp. 493-497.

[98] Zoarski, G.H., et al., Endovascular extraction of malpositioned fibered platinum microcoils from the aneurysm sac during endovascular therapy. American Journal of Neuroradiology, 1997. **18**(4): pp. 691-695.

[99] Prestigiacomo, C.J., K. Fidlow, and J. Pile-Spellman, Retrieval of a fractured Guglielmi detachable coil with use of the Goose Neck snare "twist" technique. Journal of Vascular and Interventional Radiology, 1999. **10**(9): pp. 1243-1247.

[100] Eeckhout, E., J.C. Stauffer, and J.J. Goy, Retrieval of a migrated coronary stent by means of an alligator forceps catheter. Catheterization and Cardiovascular Interventions, 1993. **30**(2): pp. 166-168.

[101] Byrne, J., et al., A novel flexible endovascular stent for use in small and tortuous vessels. Neuroradiology, 2000. **42**(1): pp. 56-61.

[102] Gill, K.S. and R.C. Fowler, Atherosclerotic renal arterial stenosis: clinical outcomes of stent placement for hypertension and renal failure. Radiology, 2003. **226**(3): pp. 821-826.

[103] Slonim, S.M., et al., Management of misplaced or migrated endovascular stents. Journal of Vascular and Interventional Radiology, 1999. **10**(7): pp. 851-859.

[104] Koseoglu, K., et al., Retrieval of intravascular foreign bodies with goose neck snare. European Journal of Radiology, 2004. **49**(3): pp. 281-285.

[105] Laganà, D., et al., Multimodal approach to endovascular treatment of visceral artery aneurysms and pseudoaneurysms. European Journal of Radiology, 2006. **59**(1): pp. 104-111.

[106] Kasirajan, K., et al., Chronic mesenteric ischemia: open surgery versus percutaneous angioplasty and stenting. Journal of Vascular Surgery, 2001. **33**(1): pp. 63-71.

[107] Cognet, F., et al., Chronic mesenteric ischemia: Imaging and percutaneous treatment 1. Radiographics, 2002. **22**(4): pp. 863-879.

[108] Lee, J.T., et al., Stent-graft migration following endovascular repair of aneurysms with large proximal necks: anatomical risk factors and long-term sequelae. Journal of Endovascular Therapy, 2002. **9**(5): pp. 652-664.

[109] Resch, T., et al., Distal migration of stent-grafts after endovascular repair of abdominal aortic aneurysms. Journal of Vascular and Interventional Radiology, 1999. **10**(3): pp. 257-264.

[110] Schütz, A., et al., Proximal stent fixation of fractured coils: technical note. Neuroradiology, 2005. **47**(11): pp. 874-878.

[111] Fiorella, D., et al., Monorail snare technique for the recovery of stretched platinum coils: technical case report. Neurosurgery, 2005. **57**(1): p. E210.

[112] Udd, M., et al., Treatment of bleeding pseudoaneurysms in patients with chronic pancreatitis. World Journal of Surgery, 2007. **31**(3): pp. 504-510.

[113] Tisnado, J., et al., Peripheral embolization of a stainless steel coil. American Journal of Roentgenology, 1979. **133**(2): pp. 324-326.

[114] Bendszus, M., et al., Neurologic complications after particle embolization of intracranial meningiomas. American Journal of Neuroradiology, 2005. **26**(6): pp. 1413-1419.

[115] Makuuchi, M., et al., Bile duct necrosis: complication of transcatheter hepatic arterial embolization. Radiology, 1985. **156**(2): pp. 331-334.

[116] Mehta, R.I., et al., Hydrophilic polymer emboli: an under-recognized iatrogenic cause of ischemia and infarct. Modern Pathology, 2010. **23**(7): pp. 921-930.

[117] Shannon, P., et al., Inadvertent foreign body embolization in diagnostic and therapeutic cerebral angiography. American Journal of Neuroradiology, 2006. **27**(2): p. 278-282.

[118] Raftopoulos, C., et al., Transvascular coil hooking procedure to retrieve an unraveled Guglielmi detachable coil: technical note. Neurosurgery, 2002. **50**(4): pp. 912-915.

[119] Henkes, H., et al., Endovascular coil occlusion of 1811 intracranial aneurysms: early angiographic and clinical results. Neurosurgery, 2004. **54**(2): pp. 268-285.

[120] O'Hare, A., P. Brennan, and J. Thornton, Retrieval of a migrated coil using an X6 MERCI device. Interventional Neuroradiology, 2009. **15**(1): pp. 99.

[121] Lee, C.-Y., Use of wire as a snare for endovascular retrieval of displaced or stretched coils: rescue from a technical complication. Neuroradiology, 2011. **53**(1): pp. 31-35.

[122] Leslie-Mazwi, T., et al., Stent retriever use for retrieval of displaced microcoils: a consecutive case series. American Journal of Neuroradiology, 2013. **34**(10): pp. 1996-1999.

[123] Nas, O., et al., Retrieval of a dislocated coil and stent-assisted coiling by Solitaire® stent during endovascular treatment of an intracranial aneurysm. Diagnostic and Interventional Imaging, 2016. **3**(97): pp. 381-384.

[124] Chomyn, J.J., et al., Percutaneous removal of a Gianturco coil from the pulmonary artery with use of flexible intravascular forceps. Journal of Vascular and Interventional Radiology, 1991. **2**(1): pp. 105-106.

[125] Sanchez, R.B., et al., Wallstent misplaced during transjugular placement of an intrahepatic portosystemic shunt: retrieval with a loop snare. American Journal of Roentgenology, 1992. **159**(1): pp. 129-130.

[126] Kamalesh, M., K. Stokes, and A.J. Burger, Transesophageal echocardiography assisted retrieval of embolized inferior vena cava stent. Catheterization and Cardiovascular Diagnosis, 1994. **33**(2): pp. 178-180.

[127] Bartorelli, A.L., et al., Successful transcatheter management of Palmaz Stent embolization after superior vena cava stenting. Catheterization and Cardiovascular Diagnosis, 1995. **34**(2): pp. 162-166.

[128] Grosso, M., et al., Palmaz stent dislodgement into the left pulmonary artery complicating TIPS: percutaneous retrieval and extraction after venotomy. Cardiovascular and Interventional Radiology, 1995. **18**(2): pp. 106-108.

[129] Hoyer, M.H., et al., Transcatheter retrieval of an embolized Palmaz stent from the right ventricle of a child. Catheterization and Cardiovascular Diagnosis, 1996. **39**(3): pp. 277-280.

[130] Prahlow, J.A., T.J. O'Bryant, and J.J. Barnard, Cardiac perforation due to Wallstent embolization: a fatal complication of the transjugular intrahepatic portosystemic shunt procedure. Radiology, 1997. **205**(1): pp. 170-172.

[131] Marcy, P.-Y., N. Magné, and J.-N. Bruneton, Strecker stent migration to the pulmonary artery: long-term result of a "wait-and-see attitude". European Radiology, 2001. **11**(5): pp. 767-770.

[132] ASHAR, R.M., E.A. HUETTL, and R. HALLIGAN, Percutaneous retrieval of a Wallstent from the pulmonary artery following stent migration from the iliac vein. Journal of Interventional Cardiology, 2002. **15**(2): pp. 101-106.

[133] Takahashi, T., et al., Migration of steel-wire coils into the stomach after transcatheter arterial embolization for a bleeding splenic artery pseudoaneurysm: report of a case. Surgery Today, 2001. **31**(5): pp. 458-462.

[134] Ozkan, O.S., et al., Guglielmi detachable coil erosion into the common bile duct after embolization of iatrogenic hepatic artery pseudoaneurysm. Journal of Vascular and Interventional Radiology, 2002. **13**(9): pp. 935-938.

[135] Turaga, K.K., et al., Cholangitis after coil embolization of an iatrogenic hepatic artery pseudoaneurysm: an unusual case report. Surgical Laparoscopy, Endoscopy & Percutaneous Techniques, 2006. **16**(1): pp. 36-38.

[136] Dinter, D.J., et al., Fatal coil migration into the stomach 10 years after endovascular celiac aneurysm repair. Journal of Vascular and Interventional Radiology, 2007. **18**(1): pp. 117-120.

[137] Reed, A., R. Suri, and R. Marcovich, Passage of embolization coil through urinary collecting system one year after embolization. Urology, 2007. **70**(6): pp. 1222. e17-1222. e18.

[138] Shah, N.A., et al., Embolization coils migrating and being passed per rectum after embolization of a splenic artery pseudoaneurysm,"the migrating coil": a case report. Cardiovascular and Interventional Radiology, 2007. **30**(6): pp. 1259-1262.

[139] Jurałowicz, P., et al., Coil migration following intravascular embolization of hepatic artery aneurysm as a cause of life-threatening obstructive jaundice-case report. Polish Journal of Surgery, 2010. **82**(12): pp. 684-686.

[140] Cishek, M.B., L. Laslett, and G. Gershony, Balloon catheter retrieval of dislodged coronary artery stents: a novel technique. Catheterization and Cardiovascular Diagnosis, 1995. **34**(4): pp. 350-352.

[141] Kiyosue, H., et al., Dispersion of coils after parent-artery occlusion of radiation-induced internal carotid artery pseudoaneurysm. American Journal of Neuroradiology, 2004. **25**(6): p. 1080-1082.

[142] Chow, M., et al., Extrusion of a coil from the internal carotid artery through the middle ear. Hong Kong Medical Journal = Xianggang yi xue za zhi/Hong Kong Academy of Medicine, 2004. **10**(3): p. 215.

[143] Dagain, A., et al., Endovascular coil transfixing a cranial nerve five years after embolisation. Acta Neurochirurgica, 2008. **150**(7): pp. 705-707.

[144] Choi, D.H., et al., Nitinol clip distal migration and resultant popliteo-tibial artery occlusion complicating access closure by the StarClose SE vascular closure system. BMJ Case Reports, 2016. **2016**: p. bcr2015012257.

[145] Sarosiek, S., M. Crowther, and J.M. Sloan, Indications, complications, and management of inferior vena cava filters: the experience in 952 patients at an academic hospital with a level I trauma center. JAMA Internal Medicine, 2013. **173**(7): pp. 513-517.

[146] Tam, M.D., et al., Fracture and distant migration of the Bard Recovery filter: a retrospective review of 363 implantations for potentially life-threatening complications. Journal of Vascular and Interventional Radiology, 2012. **23**(2):pp. 199-205. e1.

[147] Owens, C.A., et al., Intracardiac migration of inferior vena cava filters: review of published data. Chest, 2009. **136**(3): pp. 877-887.

[148] Rao, B., et al., Inferior vena cava filter-associated abnormalities: MDCT findings. AJR American Journal of Roentgenology, 2012. **198**(6): pp. W605-610.

[149] Rogers, N.A., et al., Fracture and embolization of an inferior vena cava filter strut leading to cardiac tamponade. Circulation, 2009. **119**(18): pp. 2535-2536.

[150] Taslimi R, Safari S, Kazemeini A, Aminian A, Joneidi E, Larti F. Abdominal pain due to a lost guidewire: a case report. Cases Journal. 2009;2:6680.

[151] Oh J, Kim J, Hong S, Hu C, Pyen J, Whang K, et al. Retrieval of unintended migrated detached coil: case report. The Journal of Cerebrovascular and Endovascular Neurosurgery. 2014 Sep;16(3):268-274.